Documentation Basics

A GUIDE FOR THE PHYSICAL THERAPIST ASSISTANT

Documentation Basics

A GUIDE FOR THE PHYSICAL THERAPIST ASSISTANT

Mia L. Erickson, PT, EdD, ATC, CHT
West Virginia University
Morgantown, WV

Becky McKnight, PT, MS
Ozarks Technical Community College
Springfield, MO

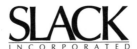

SLACK
INCORPORATED

An innovative information, education, and management company
6900 Grove Road • Thorofare, NJ 08086

www.slackbooks.com

ISBN: 978-1-55642-673-5

The procedures and practices described in this book should be implemented in a manner consistent with the professional standards set for the circumstances that apply in each specific situation. Every effort has been made to confirm the accuracy of the information presented and to correctly relate generally accepted practices. The author, editor, and publisher cannot accept responsibility for errors or exclusions or for the outcome of the application of the material presented herein. There is no expressed or implied warranty of this book or information imparted by it.

The work SLACK Incorporated publishes is peer reviewed. Prior to publication, recognized leaders in the field, educators, and clinicians provide important feedback on the concepts and content that we publish. We welcome feedback on this work.

Printed in the United States of America.

Library of Congress Cataloging-in-Publication Data

Erickson, Mia.
  Documentation basics : a guide for the physical therapist assistant / Mia Erickson, Becky McKnight.
      p. ; cm.
  Includes bibliographical references and index.
  ISBN-13: 978-1-55642-673-5 (alk. paper)
  ISBN-10: 1-55642-673-9 (alk. paper)
  1. Physical therapy assistants. 2. Physical therapy--Documentation. 3. Medical records.
  [DNLM: 1. Medical Records. 2. Physical Therapy (Specialty) 3. Allied Health Personnel.] I. McKnight, Becky. II. Title.

RM705.E74 2005
615.8'2--dc22

                                2004028539

Published by: SLACK Incorporated
                           6900 Grove Road
                           Thorofare, NJ 08086 USA
                           Telephone: 856-848-1000
                           Fax: 856-853-5991
                           www.slackbooks.com

Last digit is print number: 10   9   8   7   6   5   4   3

TABLE OF CONTENTS

An Instructor's Manual and additional materials are also available for this book from SLACK Incorporated. Don't miss these important companions to *Documentation Basics: A Guide for the Physical Therapist Assistant.* To obtain the Instructor's Manual and additional materials, please visit http://www.efacultylounge.com

ACKNOWLEDGMENTS

I would like to acknowledge the PTA Program faculty and students at Allegany College of Maryland for helping me to realize the need for this book. In addition, I would like to express my sincerest thanks to Carrie Kotlar from SLACK Incorporated for her patience throughout this process and for waiting (for a dissertation and a baby) to get the "right person" or "people" for this project. Also to Carrie, thank you for Becky! It is hard to believe that two people from different backgrounds and settings could have similar views and work ethics and work so well together. Becky, your involvement on the text and on the slides has been so encouraging. Having someone like you provided the motivation during times when I wasn't so motivated. To my husband, Jeff, not only for providing the evaluation forms in the Appendix, but also for your patience, kindness, love, and motivation. You really helped me to stay focused and encouraged me to complete this project. To my loving son, Nathan, thank you for forgiving me for the hours spent away from you and for your unconditional love. You and your father are the loves of my life. Finally, I thank God for giving me the ability to do this and for surrounding me with my support system. I know now that through You, all things are possible.

~Mia Erickson

I would like to take this opportunity to thank Dr. Loretta Knutson for identifying in me the potential for completing this project and for recommending my involvement. Also, to Mia, thank you for allowing me to "jump on board" with your dream and for giving me the opportunity to pursue mine. More importantly, I want to thank my family. To my husband, Mike, thank you for believing in me, encouraging me, and supporting me. I know being married to me is challenging at times. Thank you for your commitment to me. To my children, Crystal, Alicea, and Jessica, and my step-sons, Brett, Brantley, and Bren, thanks for putting up with all my activities and jumping in to help around the house when needed. Finally, I thank God for providing me with this opportunity. Father, thank you for continually blessing me beyond anything I could ever deserve. You have filled my life and made it overflow with riches beyond compare.

~Becky McKnight

ABOUT THE AUTHORS

Mia L. Erickson, PT, EdD, ATC, CHT

Dr. Erickson is the former Program Director of the Physical Therapist Assistant Program at Allegany College of Maryland. Currently she is an Assistant Professor and Co-Academic Coordinator of Clinical Education at West Virginia University. She has a Bachelor's Degree in Secondary Education and Athletic Training from West Virginia University and a Master of Science Degree in Physical Therapy from the University of Indianapolis. She completed her doctoral work at West Virginia University with emphasis in curriculum and instruction. She maintains clinical practice in the areas of outpatient orthopedics and hand rehabilitation.

Becky McKnight, PT, MS

Ms. McKnight is currently the Program Coordinator of the Physical Therapist Assistant Program at Ozarks Technical Community College. She received a Bachelor's Degree in Physical Therapy from St. Louis University and a post-professional Master's Degree in Physical Therapy from Rocky Mountain University of Health Professions. She has also been an Academic Coordinator of Clinical Education at Ozarks Technical Community College. She maintains clinical practice and teaching responsibilities in the areas of neurology and geriatrics.

PREFACE

Thank you for choosing *Documentation Basics: A Guide for the Physical Therapist Assistant*. Whether you are a student, a clinician, or an instructor, we believe that this book will offer you relevant, up-to-date information for surviving documentation. It is our goal for PTAs to understand their day-to-day role and to realize the importance of their documentation to Patient-Client Management.

You will notice two themes recurring throughout this text. First, we wanted to emphasize the need for relating the different aspects of the progress (or daily) notes. We believe it is important for the PTA not only to document relevant subjective information but also to relate that information to the physical therapy interventions in a way that demonstrates the role interventions play in restoring optimal function. In keeping with this theme, we also emphasize the importance of relating changes in objective data to changes in functional status.

Second, we refer to the "Physical Therapy Process" in many areas of the text. This is similar to Patient-Client Management, but it emphasizes the role of the PTA in using the physical therapist's initial examination/evaluation to structure their own interactions with patients. In other words, we guide the PTA in using the initial evaluative note to determine questions to ask, data to collect, and necessary information to document.

Chapters 1 through 3 can be used sequentially in an introductory course to set up basic rules for documenting. Chapter 4 can help answer the infamous student question, "What do I do with the patient?" Chapter 5 is designed to provide the reader with general guidelines for documentation and with specific rules for documenting patient care. While we realize the importance and need for a variety of documentation formats, it is our experience that the SOAP format is most commonly used. Therefore, we have used the SOAP structure as the basic structure for daily note writing, but emphasize the importance of function and showing relationships between each piece of the note.

For instructors and students, Chapters 6 and 7 (reimbursement and legal issues) can be used during a documentation unit or later once students have had more exposure to patient care. For practicing clinicians, Chapters 6 and 7 can provide an overview of reimbursement in different settings and important legal issues that clinicians today face. Finally, Chapter 8, SOAP Notes Across the Curriculum, can provide students with practice note writing situations for a variety of patient diagnoses and can be used in any course.

Thank you again for reviewing and using our book. Enjoy!

Physical Therapy and Disablement

Chapter One

Mia L. Erickson, PT, EdD, ATC, CHT

CHAPTER OBJECTIVES

After reading this chapter, the student will be able to:

1. Describe how the definitions of health and disability have changed throughout history.

2. Define disablement.

3. Define terminology used in the *International Classification of Functioning, Disability, and Health* (ICF) and terminology used in the Nagi framework.

4. Differentiate between impairment, functional limitation, and disability.

5. Compare and contrast the ICF and the Nagi framework.

6. Identify the relationships between impairments, functional limitations, and disabilities.

7. Differentiate between activities of daily living (ADL) and instrumental activities of daily living (IADL).

8. Define documentation.

9. Describe the relationship between documentation and disablement.

DEFINING HEALTH AND DISABILITY

A traditional approach to defining a person's "health" comes from the biomedical model in which health means free or absent from disease.[1] In this biomedical model, there is heavy emphasis on treating and curing a person's disease and little emphasis on how the disease affects the person's ability to function within society on a day-to-day basis.[1] In the 1950s and 60s, government agencies began programs to dispense funds to individuals with disabilities caused by disease or injury, eg, Social Security, Veteran's Compensation, and Worker's Compensation. However, differing definitions of disability created controversy as agencies determined the amount of money an individual was to be awarded.[2]

More contemporary models have defined "health" in terms that go beyond the patient's medical diagnosis or disease. Across the country and throughout the world, individuals and groups have developed models that acknowledge the importance of societal, psychological, and physical functioning in the presence of disease.[1] Rather than placing the measure of health on the disease process itself, more recent models have shifted toward examining an individual's ability to carry out necessary life tasks and function within society. The consequences of disease as they pertain to the relationship between body structures, ability to carry out tasks, and ability to function within society have become known as *disablement*.[3]

Today, there are 2 major disablement models, or conceptual frameworks, used to describe disability. These models include: (1) the ICF, developed by the World Health Organization (WHO), and (2) the Nagi framework, developed by Saad Nagi.

International Classification of Functioning, Disability, and Health

The ICF, originally known as the *International Classification of Impairments, Disabilities, and Handicaps* (ICIDH), was endorsed by the Fifty-Fourth World Health Assembly and released in 2001. The purpose of the ICF is to provide uniform standard language for describing health and health-related states.[4] The following definitions have been endorsed by the WHO as part of the ICF.[4]

- *Disability* encompasses impairments, activity limitations, and participation restrictions (Figure 1-1).
- An *impairment* is a problem with body function (physiological, psychological) or structure (limb, organ) such as a deviation or loss.
- *Activity limitations* are difficulties that might be encountered by an individual who is attempting to complete a task or carry out an activity.
- *Participation restrictions* are problems an individual might face while involved in life situations.

The ICF integrates the biomedical, psychological, and social aspects of diseases and their associated disabilities. Therefore, the ICF can be referred to as a "biopsychosocial model." In addition to pathophysiology of body structures and systems, the ICF takes into account the social aspects of disability and provides a mechanism to document the impact that both social and physical environments have on a person's function.[5] Using the biopsychosocial concept, the ICF describes various aspects of health as they relate to the body, the individual, and the society. This is accomplished by categorizing health information into 2 distinct but related parts: (1) Functioning and Disability and (2) Contextual Factors.[6]

Part 1, Functioning and Disability, depicts both positive (ie, function) and negative (ie, disability) aspects of health or health-related states. For example, Part 1 provides positive details on function, what the individual is able to do, regardless of his or her health. The negative aspects of health conditions are described in terms of associated body structure or system abnormalities and impairments, as well as activity limitations and participation restrictions. Part 2, Contextual Factors, comprises both environmental and personal factors that affect the individual's health and degree of disability. Environmental factors are external factors, either immediate or global, that affect the individual as he or she interacts with society. These might include physical barriers and others' opinions or attitudes. Personal factors are those that are unique to the individual, such as the ability to perform self-care skills (Figure 1-2).[6]

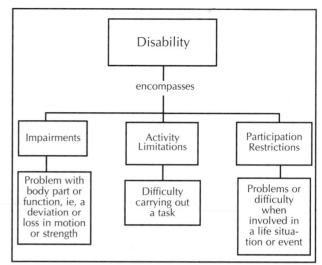

Figure 1-1. According to the World Health Organization's Model, *The International Classification of Functioning, Disability, and Health (ICF),* [4] disability encompasses an individual's impairments, activity limitations, and participation restrictions.

The ICF is part of a family of classifications created by the WHO. Its counterpart is the *International Classification of Disease, Tenth Revision* (ICD-10). The ICD-10 is a classification system for medical diagnoses and diseases, while the ICF provides a classification for function and disability for the corresponding diagnoses.[6]

The Nagi Framework

The Nagi framework was developed in the 1960s by sociologist Saad Nagi. Nagi constructed a conceptual framework using the terms active pathology, impairment, functional limitation, and disability (Figure 1-3). Nagi's model and terminology have been used in *The Guide to Physical Therapist Practice* to provide a framework for practicing therapists.[7] Nagi's model provided the following terminology and definitions.[2]

Pathology is the interruption or interference with normal process and the simultaneous body efforts to heal itself or regain a normal state. This is often referred to as the disease itself. The pathology occurs at the cellular, tissue, or organ level and is often the patient's medical diagnosis.[7] Medical management and physician interventions are often directed at reducing the active pathology. Examples of active pathologies include osteoporosis, Parkinson's disease, and fractures.

An *impairment* is a loss or abnormality of an anatomical, physiological, mental, or emotional nature. Impairments are deviations in normal anatomy or physiology. Impairments generally result from the pathology and

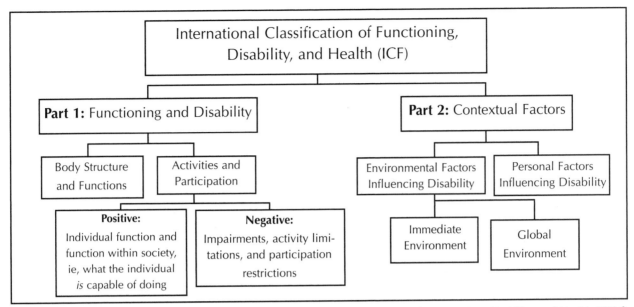

Figure 1-2. Parts of the World Health Organization's *International Classification of Functioning, Disability, and Health (ICF).*[6] Note that Part 1 includes pathophysiology as well as function in terms of what the individual can *and* can not do. Part 2 is divided into both personal and global factors that effect the degree of disability.

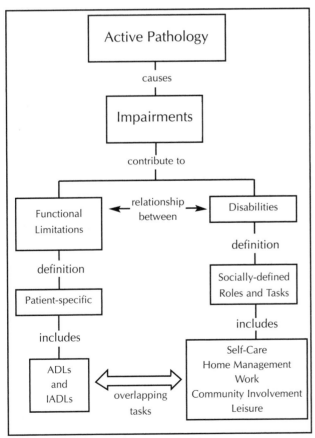

Figure 1-3. Nagi's Disablement Model.

may comprise signs and symptoms of a specific pathology. In physical therapy, common impairments include limited range of motion, muscle weakness, impaired balance, decreased sensation, and limited circulation.

A *functional limitation* refers to an abnormality or limitation in an individual's ability to carry out a meaningful action, task, or activity.[2,7] *The Guide to Physical Therapist Practice* describes 2 types of functional abilities. First, there are those associated with basic activities of daily living (ADLs), such as moving in bed, transferring from one surface to another, rising from a chair, ambulating, dressing, bathing, etc. In addition, there are activities associated with more complex independent living and community dwelling skills. These more complex behaviors are known as instrumental activities of daily living (IADLs) and include community ambulation activities, such as going to a grocery store, bank, or restaurant.[7]

Impairments often lead to functional limitations. For instance, an individual with limited shoulder range of motion (impairment) might be unable to reach into an overhead cabinet or have difficulty donning a shirt (functional limitations). While a patient with decreased quadriceps strength (impairment) might have difficulty ambulating without assistance (functional limitation). Functional limitations are patient-specific. In other words, limitations will vary depending on the individual's lifestyle and functional demands. Read the following scenarios:

- Patient 1: A 32-year-old male computer programmer with shoulder impingement syndrome has pain when reaching overhead. The patient is able to perform normal work duties since he spends most of the day at his computer.
- Patient 2: A 45-year-old male mechanic with shoulder impingement also has pain when reaching overhead. This patient is unable to work due to his inability to reach overhead since he spends most of his day with his arms in an elevated position.

In the second scenario, inability to perform normal work activities is a functional limitation, but the first patient, with the same diagnosis and chief complaint, is still able to work. Functional limitations are tasks that are specific to individual patients based on functional demands of their lifestyles and life activities.

Functional limitations relate to the fourth aspect of the Nagi framework, *disability*. The most direct way that impairments contribute to disabilities is through functional limitations.[2] According to the Nagi framework, disability is the inability or limitation in performing socially defined roles and tasks that would normally be expected of an individual within a given culture or environment.[2] Unlike functional limitations, which are patient-specific, disabilities are roles or tasks that have been socially defined as normal for a given population. These roles and tasks are organized by life activities including: (1) self-care, (2) home management, (3) work, (4) community involvement, and (5) leisure.[7]

Because disability in Nagi's model is socially constructed rather than centered on impairments or functional limitations alone, dissimilar pathologies, impairments, and functional limitations can produce similar disabilities. Furthermore, individuals with similar impairments and functional limitations might have differing degrees of disability.

The Nagi framework outlines 3 factors that influence an individual's perception of his or her degree of disability. These include: (1) the individual's situation and his or her reaction to the situation, (2) the reactions of others, such as family, friends, associates, and co-workers, and (3) environmental barriers.[2]

There is often overlap between an individual's functional limitations and his or her disabilities, and this can be a point of confusion. An individual could be limited in a task that has been determined appropriate for his or her age or environment. Let's look at an example:

- A 24-year-old male is involved in a motor vehicle accident and sustains an L2-L3 incomplete spinal cord injury. Some of his lower extremity muscles are still intact, and the patient learns to ambulate with ankle-foot orthoses and lofstrand crutches.

In this example, the individual is limited functionally due to the lower extremity weakness. He must wear assistive devices, and he probably has an abnormal gait pattern that requires high energy expenditure. Nevertheless, he can still carry out tasks that would otherwise be appropriate for a 24-year-old male; therefore, the disability, when discussing ambulation, is minimal. Now, if the same individual can only walk short distances with the assistive devices due to poor endurance and he uses a wheelchair for longer distances, the degree of disability increases. Therefore, in the latter example, the individual's disability is the inability to ambulate long distances.

PHYSICAL THERAPY AND DISABLEMENT: PUTTING IT ALL TOGETHER

Both the ICF and Nagi models provide a framework for examining the relationship between disease, impairments, functional limitations, and disability. In addition, both provide a mechanism to identify the impact of disease on an individual's day-to-day life. Consideration of a disablement model when working with patients helps therapists to realize more complex psychosocial issues that patients face. Individuals in need of physical therapy services often have a disease or injury with resulting impairments. It is our responsibility to understand how these impairments affect their day-to-day activities in a variety of settings and situations.

The physical therapy examination will illuminate the individual's impairments. These are often limitations in range of motion, strength, etc. But to see how the patient's ability to function has been compromised, the examination must go beyond the impairment level. This includes examining the patient's ability to perform things like hygiene, dressing, managing his or her home environment, and performing necessary work or school-related activities. By understanding an individual's impairments, as well as his or her life roles, we can better understand both the functional limitations and the degree of disability associated with the pathology.

The physical therapy interventions are often aimed at reducing the individual's impairments. For example, we might teach patients to perform range of motion and strengthening exercises. In doing these exercises, patients will hopefully experience decreased impairments, improved ability to function, and a reduced degree of disability.

DISABLEMENT AND DOCUMENTATION

Documentation, otherwise known as medical record-keeping, has been defined as "any entry into the patient-client record, such as a(n) consultation report, initial examination report, progress note, flow sheet/checklist, that identifies the care/service provided, re-examination, or summation of care."[7] Redgate and Foto[8] indicated that complete documentation also includes the physician prescription(s) and certification(s), communication with other care providers, copies of exercise programs or patient instructions, and any other discipline's notes or comments that support the interventions.

As you will read in subsequent chapters, documentation will serve many purposes, such as maintaining data collected on patients and providing information to insurance companies. There are also many styles and formats for physical therapy records. Regardless of the purpose and style that you are using, your documentation must reflect a disablement model. This means that physical therapy documentation should show how the patient's impairments relate to his or her limitations in function and degree of disability. Additionally, documentation should show that physical therapy interventions are bringing about substantial changes in impairment, function, and disability.

REVIEW QUESTIONS

1. How is a person's "health" determined today as opposed to 3 decades ago?

2. In your own words, describe disablement.

3. Why is there a need for disablement models today? Why are they important to you?

4. What are the 2 major disablement models today?

5. Complete the table below using terminology from the ICF and the Nagi framework. Use the following terms: pathology, impairment, functional limitation, disability, activity limitation, and participation restriction.

	IFC	Nagi
A patient's medical diagnosis		
Loss or abnormality of an individual's anatomy or physiology		
Difficulties that are encountered when an individual attempts to complete a task		
The ability to carry out a task is hindered or limited due to a problem with the anatomy or physiology		
Problems an individual faces while involved in life situations		
Encompasses impairments and limitations in abilities to carry out socially acceptable tasks		
Unable to carry out a task that would be socially appropriate for an individual		

6. What is the difference between ADL and IADL? Give 3 examples of each.

7. How are impairments and functional limitations related?

8. How are impairments, functional limitations, and disabilities related?

9. What is the role of physical therapy documentation in describing disablement?

APPLICATION EXERCISES

I.   Determine whether the following are pathology (P), impairment (I), functional limitation (FL), or disability (D) according to the Nagi framework.

   P 1. Rotator cuff tendonitis

   I 2. Decreased sensation

   I 3. Impaired balance

   P 4. Cerebrovascular accident

   FL 5. Inability to transfer out of bed

   D 6. Inability to drive without hand controls

   FL 7. Inability to rise from a chair without assistance

   P 8. Below-knee amputation

   I 9. Limited gait distance

   D 10. Inability to work

II. Of the above, which could be functional limitations and disabilities, depending on the patient? Why?

III. Read the following scenarios and determine the patient's functional limitations and disabilities.

1. You are working with a 70-year-old male who had a total hip replacement 8 weeks ago. He is now able to move in and out of the bed independently, transfer to a chair placed at the bedside, and ambulate 25 feet with a standard walker. He wants to return to driving, golfing, and playing with his grandchildren.

FL
limited gait dist.

D
Driving
golfing
playing w/ GC

2. You are working with a 10-year-old female in the school system. Her medical diagnosis (pathology) is cerebral palsy, spastic diplegia type. You have been working on ambulating up and down the stairs (which she can perform with minimum assist of 1, a quad cane, and a handrail) and increasing the speed of her gait. At the present time, she leaves her classes early so that she can make it to the next one on time, and she uses the elevator rather than the stairs.

FL
stair negotiation
decreased gait speed

D
access to school

3. Your patient is a 15-year-old who sustained a traumatic closed head injury in a motorcycle accident. He is confused and disoriented, and he requires constant supervision for his safety. He can walk and get in and out of bed with supervision. He can also ascend and descend stairs with supervision.

FL
gait
transfers
stairs

D
unable to be safe at home
or school

Chapter Two

Reasons for Documenting

Mia L. Erickson, PT, EdD, ATC, CHT

CHAPTER OBJECTIVES

After reading this chapter, the student will be able to:

1. List reasons for documenting.

2. Describe types of patient data found in a medical record.

3. Explain the "clinical decision-making process."

4. Explain the PTA's role in the clinical decision-making process.

5. Describe criteria for medical necessity and skilled care.

6. Differentiate between skilled care and maintenance therapy.

7. Realize the importance of accurate documentation.

OVERVIEW

Imagine that you are working as a PTA in a small outpatient clinic. For the last 6 weeks, you and your supervising PT have been working with a 35-year-old male who was recently involved in a motor vehicle accident. He sustained a concussion and multiple fractures including the left femur and radius. Initially, he was unable to bear weight through either extremity and required a wheelchair as his primary mode of transportation. He had significant loss in range of motion and was unable to perform self-care, home/community mobility, and work activities. He has been making excellent progress and is now able to walk using one crutch and has resumed most of his normal activities of daily living. The PT with whom you are work-ing receives a call from the patient's insurance company stating that they are going to deny payment for physical therapy services. In order to have additional therapy services approved, the clinic must submit adequate documentation showing evidence of the patient's progress.

As a PTA, documentation will be one of the most important things you do. Consider the patient case above. Continuation of his physical therapy benefits is based largely on how well the clinicians have documented his improvement. In addition to patient-related issues, like this one, there are legal, ethical, and professional obligations to maintain accurate medical records. Both state and federal laws mandate recording health care provided to an individual. In addition, maintaining accurate, timely patient records, written in a manner consistent with the *Guidelines for Physical Therapy Documentation*, is considered one of your ethical duties as a PTA. Reimbursement from third-party payers (Chapter Six) is directly linked with documentation and its ability to show the need for physical therapy services provided. In fact, the American Physical Therapy Association (APTA) House of Delegates Policy (06-94-16-28) for providing physical therapy services within the health care system states, "Reimbursement for physical therapy services should occur only when adequate physical therapy documentation exists which is consistent with APTA guidelines. Such documentation should support the need for physical therapy services."[9] Finally, facilities and organizations providing components of the patient-client management model should have policies pertaining to documentation.

In 1966, documentation became a requirement for reimbursement by government agencies such as Medicare and Medicaid. Prior to that, documentation provided a legal record of care, facilitated communication among health care providers, and served as a source of information for clinical research.[10] Shortly after that, Lawrence Weed began reporting on the use of the Problem-Oriented Medical Record (POMR). This was a type of documentation used mainly by physicians that was organized according to patient problems.

In the mid-70s, several authors reported on the use of the POMR in rehabilitation.[11-15] Reinstein et al[15] supplemented the POMR with the Rehabilitation Evaluation System that included scoring the patient's ability to perform 18 functional activities. Later they reported that this form of documentation in the rehabilitation setting improved communication among team members but was too complex for more complicated patients.[11] At about the same time, Medicare began a restructuring process and began requiring rehabilitation facilities to not only maintain documentation but also to submit the records for review by Medicare auditors. The purpose of these reviews was to determine if physical therapy services provided to Medicare beneficiaries met requirements for reimbursement. This prompted an article by Inaba and Jones,[10] which provided physical therapists with documentation requirements for reimbursement. Since then, a variety of reasons for maintaining adequate medical records, in addition to those listed above, have emerged.

REASONS FOR DOCUMENTING

Record Patient Data

One of the primary reasons for documenting physical therapy services is to maintain a record of patient data. These data should reflect the entire episode of patient care, from start to finish, beginning with an initial examination performed by the physical therapist and ending with a discharge summary. During the initial examination, the physical therapist collects and records data pertaining to the patient's current condition. This includes both subjective and objective information. Subjective information is what the patient says pertaining to his or her condition. History of the current condition, mechanism, date of onset, and history of a similar problem are all examples of subjective information gathered during the initial examination. Other subjective information collected at this point should include a thorough medical history, a review of the patient's living situation, chief complaints (including his or her functional limitations and activities that he or she is unable to complete or perform), and goals for physical therapy.

In addition to information provided by the patient about his or her condition, documented data should also include results from objective tests and measurements. Examples of these types of objective data include measurements of range of motion, strength, sensation, girth, balance, and functional status (eg, walking, transferring, and performing activities such as self-care and home management). Objective data are obtained through tests and measurements performed by the PT or through patient self-reported pain and disability questionnaires (ie, SF-36, Patient-Rated Wrist Evaluation, Oswestry Low Back Pain Disability Questionnaire). Objective data are used to examine the extent of the patient's impairments, functional limitations, and disabilities. Furthermore, these data provide us with baseline measurements to which future measurements can be compared.[16]

Record of the patient's functional status and disabilities provides particularly valuable information regarding the effects of the disease or injury on the patient's normal activities and lifestyle. Furthermore, individuals reviewing medical records deem the patient's functional status and disabilities as being more meaningful than documentation of impairments alone. While data for both impairments and function are necessary, documenting functional limitations and disabilities provides reviewers with specific contextual information regarding the impact of injury on the patient's lifestyle.

Data taken from the patient, as well as objective measurements, are not only documented during the initial examination but also during subsequent physical therapy sessions. These data are recorded in the form of progress notes or, in the case of discharge from physical therapy services, in a discharge summary. In any event, data recorded in progress and discharge notes should be compared to that in the initial examination so that the medical record reflects both subjective (patient comments) and objective (data from tests/measurements) changes in the patient's status.

Records of patient data are important to other individuals involved in the patient's care. Health care providers such as physicians, nurses, occupational and speech therapists, case managers, etc are often interested in a patient's status and therefore examine physical therapy documentation. Physicians might be interested in how far a patient can ambulate prior to deciding on discharge. Nurses might be interested in a patient's ability to transfer; whereas, case managers might want to examine equipment needs or return to work status. Therefore, documenting patient data serves as a useful tool for facilitating communication across disciplines. In addition to other health care providers, third-party payers are very interested in records of patient data. Communication with third-party payers through appropriate documentation has been determined to be the "key to securing reimbursement."[17]

Accurate records of patient data also aid in our ability to analyze and study patient outcomes. Outcomes are defined as the end result of patient-client management.[7] Collection of outcomes data is a growing area in physical therapy that is necessary for evidence-based practice. For example, analysis of patient outcomes can allow us to determine the effectiveness of physical therapy interventions. A goal of the *Guide to Physical Therapist Practice* is to standardize terminology among physical therapy providers. Use of guide-based terminology when documenting patient data can facilitate development of a national database, useful for providers who want to examine patient outcomes.[18]

Demonstrate the Clinical Decision-Making Process

From initial examination to discharge, physical therapy documentation should provide a "picture" of the clinician's decision-making process and clinical judgment.[8,19,20] Documentation that demonstrates clinical decision-making also improves the provider's credibility with third-party payers.[17] An individual who does not know the patient should be able to read the physical therapy records and identify a logical, step-wise progression from initial examination to discharge. Lewis[20] indicated that "documentation of all elements of the patient/client management model…should harmonize." Documentation should reflect logical decisions and sound judgment by showing direct links between patient problems, goals, interventions, changes in interventions, and discharge. Both the PT and PTA have specific roles in making sure this occurs:

- Data collected during the initial examination should be reflected in the plan of care. For example, goals written by the physical therapist should reflect impairments, functional limitations, and disabilities identified during the initial examination (PT role).

- The plan of care should include physical therapy interventions that are aimed at reducing the identified impairments, functional limitations, and disabilities (PT role).

- Changes in patient status should be reflected by changes in the plan of care (PT and PTA role to recognize and record changes in patient status; PTA role to communicate changes to the PT; PT role to adjust the plan of care based on patient changes).

As a PTA, you can also contribute to the decision-making process by collecting pertinent subjective and objective patient data at follow-up therapy sessions.

Subjective data often gathered and recorded by a PTA include:

- Asking the patient about his or her response to a previous treatment.

- Inquiring about compliance with a home exercise program.

- Asking the patient if the treatment has improved function.

When asking a patient if the treatment has improved function, it is important to refer back to the initial evaluation to see what limitations the patient had when he or she started the episode of care. That way, you can be specific in your inquiries.

Prior to collecting objective data through tests and measurements, it is important to see what measurements were taken during the initial evaluation. That way, you have a baseline to which your measurements can be compared. In addition, it is important to try to speak with the PT about the patient prior to the treatment session. At that time you can ask whether or not certain tests and measurements are needed.

Objective data often gathered by a PTA include:
- Goniometric measurements
- Manual muscle testing
- Functional status (bed mobility, transfers, gait)

PTAs should record subjective patient comments and results of relevant tests and measurements in progress notes or updates. These progress notes serve to reveal changes in impairments, functional limitations, and disabilities that were found during the initial examination. Findings that warrant re-evaluation, changes in the plan of care, or discharge should also be provided in the documentation and communicated to the PT.

When there is consistency between the initial examination and progress notes, the clinical decision-making process is easily identified. Documentation of subjective remarks and objective findings begins to tell the story of the patient's response to therapy. In addition, consistency between initial and subsequent documentation makes it easier for the clinician(s) to identify progress, or lack thereof. Finally, using data gathered during the initial examination allows the PT to easily update goals and interventions as needed. This "process" will be described in more detail in Chapter Four.

Provide Proof of Medical Necessity

Our documentation must provide evidence that physical therapy services are *both* medically necessary *and* require skills of trained personnel (otherwise known as skilled care). The Centers for Medicare & Medicaid Services[21] has defined medically necessary as services or supplies that:

1. Are appropriate and needed for the diagnosis or treatment of a medical condition.

2. Are provided for the diagnosis, direct care, and treatment of a medical condition.

3. Meet the standards of good medical practice in the local area.

4. Are not mainly for the convenience of the patient or health care provider.

Determination of whether an intervention is medically necessary is based on our knowledge of the patient's pathology (or disease process), familiarity with physical therapy interventions and their alternatives, and awareness of the standards of practice for treating that pathology.[22] In proving medical necessity, documentation from the initial examination must demonstrate how the patient's pathology has caused functional limitations and disabilities and must outline a specific plan of care that will address these limitations. In addition, the patient should have good potential for meeting the goals set by the physical therapist, such that achieving functional gains occurs within a reasonable amount of time.

In most cases, medical necessity is initially established by the referring physician or physical therapist; nevertheless, it is important for a PTA to recognize when the intervention is no longer medically necessary. Intervention may no longer be medically necessary if: (1) the patient has met all the goals that have been established by the physical therapist, (2) the patient is no longer benefiting from the intervention, or (3) the services can be carried out through home exercise instructions or by untrained personnel. Treatment might also exceed criteria for medical necessity if the patient, family, or caregiver(s) has unrealistic expectations for recovery.[8]

Documentation showing objective, comparative data, as well as functional limitations and improvements, can provide evidence that a patient is progressing toward the goals stated in the plan of care. Documentation can then further support the need for subsequent or continued interventions due to medical necessity, or it can provide a rationale for discontinuing physical therapy services.

Provide Proof of Skilled Care

In addition to proving that treatments are medically necessary, documentation must reflect the patient's need for skilled care. Skilled care, otherwise known as skilled services, has been defined as a type of health care given when a patient needs management, observation, or evaluation by trained nurses or rehabilitation staff.[21] In order for a physical therapy intervention to be considered "skilled," a patient must have a pathology or injury that results in a documented physical or functional limitation and requires a sophisticated and complex intervention that can only be carried out by a licensed PT or PTA. This intervention requires the unique judgment and skill of a trained individual for both safety and effectiveness. In addition, the intervention must be both reasonable and medically necessary, and it must reflect the accepted standard of practice. Skilled interventions have been proven safe, effective, and specific to the patient's condition. Finally, improvement in the patient's condition should be expected within a reasonable and predictable amount of time.[8]

Services that are not considered skilled care are often known as "maintenance" therapy. Maintenance therapy services can be provided by a non-licensed individual, such as a family member or caregiver who has had some training from a skilled professional, or by the patient through independent home exercises. Maintenance services are not reimbursed by Medicare or many other third-party payers.[22]

The Event of Legal Action

Medical records are legal documents, and any entry you make into the medical record becomes part of that legal document. For this reason, it is important your documentation is accurate, legible, and that it depicts the patient's condition and the intervention appropriately and completely. Be aware that a patient's medical records can be subpoenaed and used as evidence in a variety of legal matters. These include motor vehicle accidents, worker's compensation or disability claims, and malpractice suits brought against you or other health care providers.

In malpractice lawsuits, documentation is the clinician's first line of defense. Good documentation can stop a lawsuit in its tracks, and poor documentation can be "powerful evidence in support of a suit, even when the accusations are frivolous."[20] Consider the following as a rule of thumb: "If it isn't documented, it didn't happen." Following the guidelines for documentation in this text, recommendations set forth by the APTA, state and federal laws, government agencies' regulations (ie, Medicare and Medicaid), and facility policies can help to protect you if you become involved in a malpractice lawsuit.

REVIEW QUESTIONS

1. List reasons for documenting.

2. How can a PTA demonstrate the clinical decision-making process in his or her documentation?

3. What are examples of subjective and objective data that can be gathered by a PTA?

4. What are the criteria for determining if a treatment or intervention is medically necessary?

5. Who determines medical necessity initially?

6. What is the difference between skilled care and maintenance therapy? Provide an example of each.

7. What is the role of the PTA in determining medical necessity?

8. How does the patient's rehabilitation potential influence his or her need for medically necessary skilled care?

9. Review the *Guide for Conduct of the Physical Therapist Assistant* (www.apta.org), and identify your professional obligation(s) that pertain to documentation.

APPLICATION EXERCISES

I.   Read through the following examination/evaluation and answer the questions that follow.

Date: March 15, 2004

Pr: 27 y.o. ♂ s/p (L) wrist and ankle fx; Begin gentle wrist and ankle AROM & PROM; May begin using cx c̄ platform for (L) UE. PWB 50% on (L) LE

S: *HPI:* 4 weeks s/p fall (~25') from a logging truck landing on his (L) side (2/1/04). Pt. sustained fx of the (L) distal radius and ulna and (L) distal tibia and fibula. Pt. underwent ORIF for the wrist and ankle immediately p̄ the injury. He was placed in a SAC for the UE and SLC for the LE. He was NWB on the (L) LE and has been unable to use cx 2° to not being allowed to bear weight on the affected UE. At the time of the fall, the pt. also sustained a mild concussion. He was hospitalized for 5 days following the injury. While hospitalized he received IP PT to learn how to negotiate his w/c and perform transfers. Both casts were removed yesterday and his ankle was placed in a removable splint. Reports taking ibuprofen PRN for pain.

   C/C: Pain and stiffness in (L) UE & LE c̄ ↓functional use of (B). Doesn't like using w/c for mobility. Unable to work. Requiring assist c̄ self-care activities and home management.

   L/S: RHD; Lives c̄ wife and 2 small children in single level home c̄ 2 steps @ entrance c̄ HR on the (R). Prior to injury pt. was employed as a construction worker. He has been off work since the DOI. Pt. is unable to drive and is relying on his wife & mother for transportation. No significant PMH or hx of fx. Reports being a non smoker and non-drinker. Family hx is (+) for OA.

   Pt's Goals: Return to previous level of function and RTW ASAP. Learn to ambulate with cx.

O: *AROM:* (R) UE & LE WNL; (L) shoulder, elbow, & hip WNL

		AROM	PROM
(L) wrist:			
	Flexion	20°	25°
	Extension	10°	15°
	UD	10°	15°
	RD	15°	15°
	Supination	30°	35°
	Pronation	40°	45°

   (L) hand: Pt. can perform a full fist but it is difficult 2° to edema. Thumb IP, MCP, and CMC AROM is WNL

(L) knee:		0-100°	0-110°
(L) ankle:			
	DF	-10°	-5°
	PF	20°	25°
	Inv	5°	5°
	Ev	0°	5°

   Strength: (R) UE & LE 5/5; (L) shoulder and hip 4/5; (L) elbow, wrist, knee, & ankle deferred 2° to acuity

   Girth: wrist figure 8 (R): 36 cm (L): 37.2 cm; ankle figure 8 (R): 42 cm (L): 44.1 cm

   Sensation: (L) wrist and ankle intact to light touch & (=) when compared to (R)

   Circulation: 2+ at radial & dorsal pedal arteries on the (L)

   Special Tests: N/A @ this time 2° to acuity

   Gait: Unable to ambulate at this time

   Transfers: (I) bed ↔ chair, chair ↔ toilet, sit ↔ stand all NWB on (L) LE

   Bed Mobility: (I) all areas.

   Tx & HEP: AROM & PROM for (L) wrist for flexion, extension, pronation, & supination and for (L) ankle DF and PF, used opposite foot for self PROM of ankle; performed AROM for all digits and thumb; initiated compression glove for edema to be worn n.s.; instructed pt. in elevation and compression wrapping for ankle and wrist; instructed pt. in use of cx with platform for (L) UE PWB 50% (L) using step to gait pattern. Pt. required CGA x 1 for balance. The pt. performed all ex. (I) and verbalized understanding of all precautions.

A: 27 y.o. RHD ♂ 4 wks s/p fall where he sustained fx to the (L) wrist & ankle. Now c̄ ↓ AROM, PROM, and strength. Inability to ambulate, perform self-care, or home management tasks s̄ assistance. Unable to work @ this time. Skilled services necessary to instruct pt. in appropriate ROM ex., use of AD & progress gait as ordered. Also will require instruction in strengthening exercises and retraining in functional mobility to prepare for return to normal L/S and RTW. Pt. able to communicate s̄ limitations and demonstrates excellent motivation and good potential for full recovery. No co-morbidities that could affect outcome identified at this time.

        Anticipated Goals and Expected Outcomes:

- At the end of 2 weeks, the pt. will:
  1.   Increase AROM 10-15° for the wrist, forearm, and ankle
  2.   Decrease edema by .5 cm for the wrist and ankle
  3.   Ambulate c̄ cx c̄ (L) UE platform PWB (L) LE (I)
  4.   Perform all self-care (I)
  5.   Perform a full fist s̄ limitations
- At the end of 16 weeks (d/c), the pt. will:
  1.   Have normal AROM of the wrist, forearm, and ankle (90-100% of opposite)
  2.   Grip and pinch strength will be 80-100% of (R)
  3.   Be (I) c̄ all self-care & home management tasks
  4.   Ambulate (I) on all surfaces s̄ use of AD
  5.   ↑↓flight of stairs (I) s̄ AD
  6.   Drive s̄ restrictions
  7.   RTW @ previous level of employment

P: See pt. 3x/wk for next 3-4 mos. to work on AROM & PROM of the wrist and ankle; general LE ex. for the hip, knee, shoulder, and elbow; gait training; functional mobility; & strengthening to involved joints when appropriate. Will progress pt. as tolerated & according to MD orders. Pt. is in agreement c̄ the above stated plan.

                                                   John Smith, PT

1. List 5 of the patient's impairments.

   ↓ AROM wrist, ankle, knee Ⓛ   ↓ WB Ⓛ LE
   ↓ strength Ⓛ shld + hip
   ↑ girth
   pain

2. List 5 of the patient's functional (activity) limitations and particpation restrictions.

   Ø gait   unable to drive
   Ø self-care
   Ø home management
   Ø stairs

3. Is this patient disabled? Why or why not?

   Unable to access home I + unable to work

4. In this example, how are the patient's impairments creating functional limitations and disability?

5. List 5 pieces of subjective data found in the evaluation.

① UE & LE pain /stiff   Requiring A
Doesn't like w/c   unable to work
home set up
pt goals

6. List 5 pieces of objective data found in the evaluation.

ROM
MMT
girth
Sensation
mobility

7. How did the PT describe the need for skilled care?

8. What information would you need to provide in a progress note for this patient to show medical necessity and the need for further skilled care?

9. Is this patient's care medically necessary? Why or why not? What evidence is there of medical necessity?

10. What other providers/individuals might be interested in looking at this patient's note(s)?

II. Read through the following scenarios, and decide if the treatment would be considered maintenance or skilled. Give an explanation for your answer. If you choose maintenance, what are some things that you should do (as a PTA) to discontinue treatment?

1. You are working with a patient in a nursing home who has severe Alzheimer's disease. Every afternoon, you take her for a walk through the hallways around the building. She demonstrates weakness in her right ankle, and there is a foot slap during the contact phase of gait. She can control it if given verbal cuing. You have been working with her for a month. You are not seeing any follow-through from one session to the next, and she has not progressed her distance in the last 2 weeks.

M

2. You have been working for a home health agency in the evenings to make some extra money. The patient you are currently seeing has not shown improvement in the last week. She is an 85-year-old lady with Parkinson's disease who lives with her daughter. You are considering recommending discharge when one day the patient's daughter tells you that her mother enjoys having you come in, and they really believe that you are helping.

M - S

3. You are working in a skilled nursing unit, and you are assigned a patient who requires maximum assist for transfers and can not participate in therapy due to lethargy and confusion. Every day you do PROM to all extremities and transfer the patient to the bedside chair.

M

4. You and your supervising PT are working in an outpatient physical therapy clinic with a patient who has a frozen shoulder. She has been participating in therapy for about 6 weeks. During that time she has made a substantial amount of progress. Recently her ROM has started to plateau. The patient attends therapy twice a week for stretching and joint mobilizations.

S

5. You are working on gait training with a patient who had a right CVA and has resultant left hemiplegia. While ambulating, you provide tactile and verbal cuing to the quadriceps to achieve full knee extension in late swing. The patient can respond to your cues about 50% of the time. Gait has improved over the last week.

S

Chapter Three

Documentation Formats

Mia L. Erickson, PT, EdD, ATC, CHT

CHAPTER OBJECTIVES

After reading this chapter, the student will be able to:

1. List 4 types of documentation formats used in physical therapy.

2. Examine different types of physical therapy documentation formats.

3. Describe each type of documentation.

4. Explain advantages and disadvantages of different documentation formats including narrative and SOAP notes, problem-oriented medical records (POMR), and functional outcomes reporting (FOR).

5. Differentiate between information found in the S, O, A, and P portions of a SOAP note.

6. Identify positive and negative aspects of using forms and templates.

7. Examine positive and negative aspects of computerized documentation.

Documentation in physical therapy practice can take on a variety of formats depending on the type of patients being treated, practice setting, state laws and practice acts, and reimbursement requirements. Different documentation formats include: narrative reports, problem-oriented medical records (POMR), SOAP, and functional outcomes reporting (FOR) (Figure 3-1). A brief discussion of each of these formats is provided in this chapter.

NARRATIVE

In narrative documentation, the clinician describes the patient encounter. This type of documentation provides pertinent information written mainly in paragraph format. There may or may not be headings identifying important information. Headings used in narrative notes are at the discretion of the clinician writing the note. When using the narrative format, Quinn and Gordon[3] recommend that you develop an outline of information to cover so that important details are not omitted.

Narrative Example:

Date: 3/3/04

Patient: John Smith

Pt. RTC reporting no adverse effects from tx last visit or from HEP. He stated that he feels as though his wrist & ankle are moving a little better and the edema in the hand has ↓. He reports that he is able to shower (I) using a plastic chair in the tub and feels like he has improved c̄ his ability to dress himself. AROM of the (L) wrist is as follows: flexion 30°, extension 30°, UD 15°, RD 20°, supination 45°, and pronation 60°; (L) knee: 0-135°; (L) ankle DF-PF 5-45°. Figure 8 wrist girth is 35.5 cm and ankle figure 8 girth is 43 cm on the (L). Pt. is ambulating household distances (I) c̄ cx using (L) UE platform, PWB 50% on the (L) LE. (I) with all

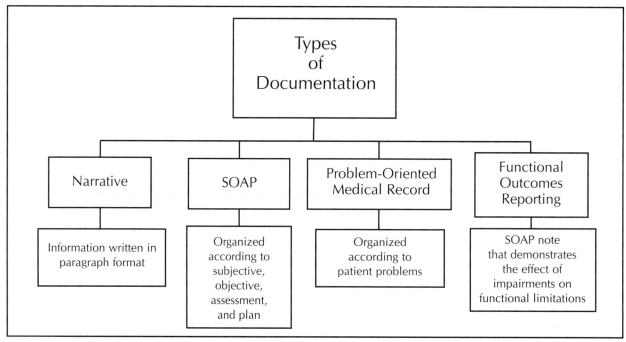

Figure 3-1. Types of documentation used in physical therapy.

transfers and self-care. Tx consisted of gentle AROM and PROM for 30' to the (L) wrist and forearm in the directions of flexion, extension, supination, & pronation, and to the (L) ankle for DF, PF, inv, & ev. Pt. also performed AROM for the hand. The pt. has made improvements in AROM and has ↓ edema. Improvements have allowed pt. to improve his ability to ambulate (I) and perform self-care. Will continue to have the pt. perform his HEP and RTC on 3/5/04.

Bill Jones, PTA

There are times when the narrative format is the most appropriate format to use. These include describing a sequence of events, brief interactions with patients, conversations with other health care providers, or any other situation that requires a detailed explanation and none of the other documentation formats are appropriate. In these instances, you can simply describe the situation and how it affects the patient in a brief narrative note. Narrative notes are sometimes the easiest to use when you just need to describe the details of a situation and you are trying to paint a vivid description of what happened.

Example:
Date: 6/18/03
Patient: John Smith
Spoke with patient's physician today regarding the amount of weight bearing he is allowed to perform when ambulating with the platform cx. He stated that his fx sites on the radius and ulna are stable and healing well, and he can WBAT on the UE. Will have patient continue to use crutches with platform on the (L), allowing him to weight bear through the extremity as indicated by the physician.

Authors have identified several problems with the narrative record. First, due to the lack of structure, the writer is prone to omit details that could potentially be very important. In addition, there is a high degree of variability among clinicians.[3] When medical notes are lacking structure, it might be very difficult to read and locate necessary information. For example, it would be very time consuming for a case manager to sort through a chart filled with unstructured narrative entries to locate information regarding the patient's ability to transfer. Furthermore, following the clinician's problem-solving process can be difficult in narrative reports.[24] For these reasons, more structured documentation formats have emerged.

PROBLEM-ORIENTED MEDICAL RECORD

The problem-oriented medical record (POMR) was introduced by Lawrence Weed to provide medical students with a structured documentation format oriented around the patient's problems.[24] He believed that the narrative format was often confusing and unorganized, making it difficult to determine how the physician defined and treated various patient problems.[24] In the POMR, the first page consists of a patient-problem list. This serves as the "Table of Contents" for the remainder of the medical record.

Example:

Problem #1: ↓ A/PROM left wrist

Problem #2: ↓ A/PROM left ankle

Problem #3: ↓ strength left wrist

Problem #4: ↓ strength left ankle

Problem #5: ↓ (I) c̄ ambulation

Subsequent entries, or progress notes, are organized according to these problems. For each entry, the physician discusses management of each problem in the following terms:

- *Subjective Data:* This includes symptomatic data provided by the patient.
- *Objective Data:* Identifies results of tests and measurements performed or physical exam data.
- *Impression (Imp.):* The practitioner's impression of the patient and that particular problem.
- *Treatment and Therapy (Rx):* Treatment or therapy provided for that particular problem on that day or during that session.
- *Immediate Plans (Plan):* Treatment plan for that particular problem.

Example:

Problem #1: ↓ A/PROM left wrist
Subj: Pt. reports no adverse effects from last treatment; States that the wrist and hand are moving better allowing him improved functional activities
Obj: AROM (L) wrist: flexion 30°, extension 30°, UD 15°, RD 20°, supination 45°, and pronation 60°
Imp: A/PROM improving with exercise; improvements allowing more functional use of the wrist and hand
Rx: 2 x 10 reps AROM and PROM for flexion, extension, supination, and pronation
Plan: Have pt. continue c̄ HEP and RTC in 2 days

Using this format, the reader can identify the patient's care for each of the identified problems.

Major advantages of POMR include:[11-13,25,26]

1. Provides organization and structure to the medical information.

2. Includes a comprehensive list of the patient's problems.

3. Discusses each of the patient's problems separately.

4. Provides a specific plan for managing each of the patient's problems (ie, treatment is problem-oriented).

5. Allows a physician who is interested in a particular problem to go directly to that aspect of the note, thus improving communication among care providers.

6. Provides a chronological sequence of interventions for a particular problem, better outlining the problem-solving process.

Regardless of the benefits to the structure provided with the POMR, authors have reported problems with it as well. First, the POMR separates, or fragments, patients according to their problems, and this might pose a problem in complex cases if a provider doesn't see the "whole patient."[25] In the case of John Smith, it is possible that a therapist working with the upper extremity might not be aware of the lower extremity problems without reading separate chart entries. This could be very time consuming. In addition, for patients with multiple problems, the POMR can become increasingly complex, requiring an extraordinary amount of time for an individual managing multiple problems. In our example, the patient has many problems, and for one therapist, this could result in as many as 5 to 6 different chart entries per visit. Therefore, it is not suitable for more complex rehabilitation patients.[11]

SOAP Notes

SOAP is an acronym for Subjective, Objective, Assessment, and Plan. SOAP evolved from the POMR documentation format initially provided by Weed as described in the preceding section. Like with the POMR, "S," or subjective, should include anything the patient tells you pertaining to his or her injuries or problems. Subjective information can also be any information provided by the patient's family or caregivers. The "O," or objective, section should include relevant tests and measurements performed, the patient's functional status, and physical therapy interventions performed for that day of service. Unlike the POMR, in the SOAP format, the physical therapy interventions are written in the objective portion of the note. The interpretation, or impression, has been designated "A," for assessment. In SOAP format, the "P" stands for plan. More detailed examples of information provided in the S, O, A, and P portions of the notes can be found in Figures 3-2 through 3-5.

Unlike the POMR, one SOAP note generally includes information pertaining to all of the patient's problems. However, the SOAP note may or may not be preceded by a problem ("Pr") section. When it is, the "Pr" section contains information pertaining to the medical diagnosis

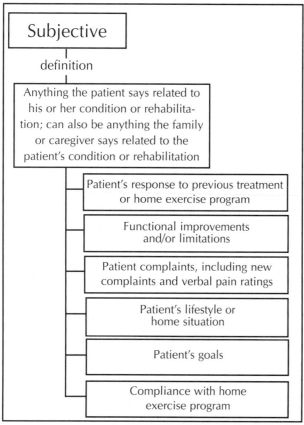

Figure 3-2. Information included in the "S" (Subjective) portion of the note.

and/or referral information (example below). You will read more about the SOAP sections, including the problem section, in Chapter 4.

The SOAP format is now widely used by a variety of medical and rehabilitation professionals, although it is no longer associated with the POMR.[3] SOAP has become a stand-alone format for documentation. Like the POMR, SOAP note documentation provides structure to medical record entries and should be used to show logical decision-making by using subjective and objective information to determine an assessment and plan.

SOAP Example:
(*Please note*: This is the same information that was provided in the narrative and POMR notes above. Pay particular attention to the organization of subjective and objective information as well as the assessment and plan under the appropriate headings):

Date: 3/3/04

Pr: 27 y.o. ♂ s/p (L) wrist and ankle fx; Begin gentle wrist and ankle AROM & PROM

S: Pt. RTC reporting no adverse effects from tx last visit or from HEP. He stated that his wrist & ankle are moving a little better and the edema in the hand has ↓. He reports that he is able to shower (I) using a plastic chair in the tub and feels like he has improved c̄ his ability to dress himself.

O: *AROM* (L) wrist: flexion 30°, extension 30°, UD 15°, RD 20°, supination 45°, pronation 60°; (L)

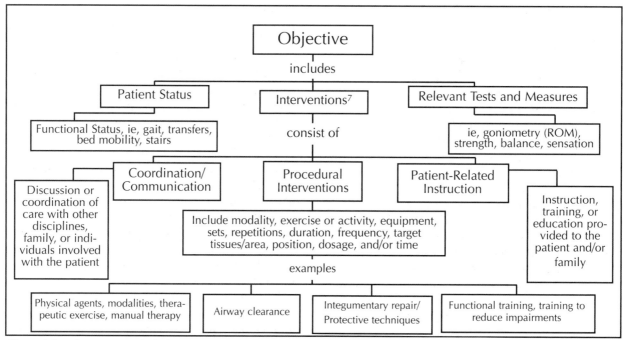

Figure 3-3. Information included in the "O" (Objective) portion of the note.

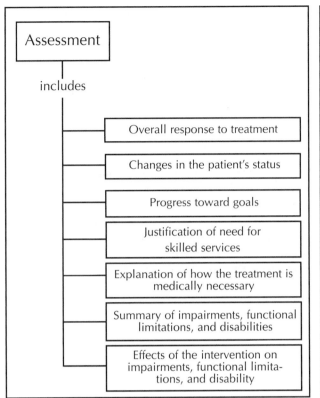

Figure 3-4. Information included in the "A" (Assessment) portion of the note.

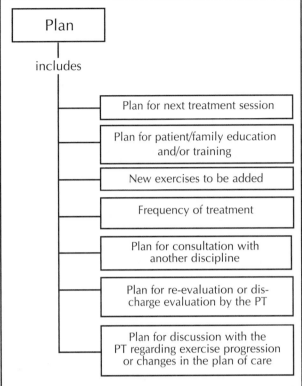

Figure 3-5. Information included in the "P" (Plan) portion of the note.

knee: 0-135°; (L) ankle DF-PF 5-45°. *Girth:* (L) wrist figure 8: 35.5 cm and (L) ankle figure 8: 43 cm. *Tx:* gentle AROM and PROM for 30' to the (L) wrist & forearm for flexion, extension, supination, & pronation. Pt. also performed hand AROM. **A:** The pt. has made improvements in AROM and has ↓ edema. Improvements have allowed pt. to improve ability to ambulate (I) and perform self-care.
P: Will continue to have the pt. perform his HEP and RTC on 3/5/04.

Bill Jones, PTA

Even though SOAP notes provide a consistent and concise format for documenting the patient's subjective remarks, objective exam findings, the provider's overall impression, and the plan of care, the documentation procedure has been scrutinized recently. Several reasons for this scrutiny exist. First, objective findings are often written in terms of impairments, such as range of motion, strength, balance, etc. Furthermore, links between improvements in the patient's impairments and improved functional capabilities are usually implied, rather than described in detail.[27,28] This often results in documentation centered around the patient's complaints and impairments, rather than documentation that focuses on progress and improving function. In addition, SOAP notes usually don't show how the interventions are contributing to functional improvements. Nevertheless, the SOAP format is widely accepted and can be an appropriate form of documentation if its emphasis shifts toward linking impairment, function, and intervention.

FUNCTIONAL OUTCOMES REPORTING (FOR)

Functional outcomes reporting (FOR) is becoming more popular in rehabilitation. Quinn and Gordon[3] describe FOR as a type of documentation that focuses on the ability to perform meaningful functional activities rather than concentrating on isolated musculoskeletal, neuromuscular, cardiopulmonary, or integumentary impairments. Advantages of FOR have been identified. FOR establishes a relationship between the patient's impairments and the ability to perform functional tasks, and it improves readability for non-health care providers reviewing documentation.[3,29]

While the importance of FOR has been provided in preceding sections, SOAP format is still the most common type of documentation used in physical therapy practice.

Authors have suggested combining FOR with the SOAP format.[29,30] When combining FOR with the SOAP format, Abeln[29] suggested making the following additions to SOAP:

1. Objective (O) Section: Clearly and objectively describe the patient's functional status, including functional activities that are specific to that patient.

2. Assessment (A) Section: List only those impairments being addressed with therapy. Describe how improvement in impairments will lead to improvement in functional limitations. Provide complicating factors, ie, co-morbidities. PTs write goals using functional terminology.

Example (SOAP and FOR Combined):

(*Please note*: The following is the same example that was used to demonstrate narrative, POMR, and SOAP formats. This example combines the FOR with the SOAP format as recommended by Abeln.[29] Additions are presented in *italics*.)

Date: 3/3/04

S: Pt. RTC reporting no adverse effects from tx last visit or from HEP. He stated that his wrist & ankle are moving a little better and the edema in the hand has ↓. He reports that he is able to shower (I) using a plastic chair in the tub and feels like he has improved c̄ his ability to dress himself.

O: *AROM* (L) wrist: flexion 30°, extension 30°, UD 15°, RD 20°, supination 45°, pronation 60°; (L) knee: 0-135°; (L) ankle DF-PF 5-45°. *Girth*: (L) wrist figure 8: 35.5 cm and (L) ankle figure 8: 43 cm. *Functional Status*: Gait: *Ambulates household distances with (B) axillary cx c̄ (L) UE platform, PWB 50% (L), (I).* Transfers: *(I) c̄ all transfers* Self-care: *(I) c̄ showering and dressing.* IADLs: *Unable to work; Unable to assist wife c̄ child care duties.* Tx: gentle AROM and PROM for 30' to the (L) wrist & forearm for flexion, extension, supination, & pronation. Pt. also performed hand AROM.

A: The pt. has made improvements in AROM and has ↓ edema, *although both remain to be impairments. Decreased edema and exercise have improved AROM allowing improved use of wrist & hand during self-care and use of ankle for normal gait pattern. Continues to require use of cx 2° to PWB status—this is limiting his ability to ambulate s̄ an AD.*

P: Will continue to have the pt. perform his HEP and RTC on 3/5/04.

Bill Jones, PTA

This chapter outlines several different types of physical therapy notes, each being used to document patient care. These included the narrative note, POMR, SOAP notes, and FOR. In hospitals and clinical settings, you are likely to encounter a wide variety of documentation formats, and it is important that you adhere to both state and federal laws as well as your facility's approved format. It is the author's experience that the POMR is least prevalent while the SOAP format is most widely used; however, FOR is becoming increasingly more popular. Narrative notes also serve distinct purposes as previously described. Although there is no documented evidence suggesting superiority of one type of note over another, you will soon find that in real-world clinical practice, you are likely to apply principles from the 3 latter types, thus using a combination of narrative, SOAP, and FOR. The authors of this text have selected the SOAP format to provide a framework for basic documentation skills. This format was selected because of its prevalence in clinical practice and because of its adaptability to a variety of documentation styles, thus meeting the needs of your employer and payer sources, and complying with the law. In this text, you will learn to use SOAP as the basic structure for your notes. However, additional emphasis will be placed on documenting the patient's functional status; linking impairments, functional limitations, and interventions; linking interventions with improvement; and referring to the initial evaluative note for making clinical decisions.

TEMPLATES AND FILL-IN FORMS

In order to facilitate documentation and eliminate time constraints, clinicians have started using a variety of documentation templates and fill-in forms. Forms can be either paper or computer-based. These forms not only save time but have potential to minimize writing, improve accuracy and consistency across patients, prompt clinicians to provide more data,[31] and include essential documentation requirements set forth by Medicare or other third-party payers.[32] Initial evaluations, progress notes, reevaluations, discharge summaries, and physician progress updates are often written using standard forms developed by individual facilities. Several paper examples of standardized forms and templates have been provided in Appendix B. *The Guide to Physical Therapy Practice* also includes documentation templates for both inpatient and outpatient physical therapy.[7]

Forms and templates can also provide a mechanism for multidisciplinary documentation in which each discipline has its own section to complete on the same form. For example, in inpatient rehabilitation settings and in skilled nursing facilities, Medicare payment is determined by data provided through multidisciplinary fill-in forms. Examples of multidisciplinary forms include the Minimum Data Set, used in skilled nursing facilities, and the Inpatient Rehabilitation Facility Patient Assessment Instrument, used in inpatient rehabilitation hospitals.

While fill-in forms and templates often ease time constraints and improve consistency, both PTs and PTAs must take care in not allowing the form to "dictate" the session. This is especially important for students and new graduates who may feel like they can not deviate from the form. In some instances, clinical instructors and employers will require students and new graduates to document using one of the above described formats (Narrative, SOAP, etc) rather than using the standard facility templates or fill-in forms. More importantly though, forms can promote incomplete documentation.[20,33] Providers must be sure that forms contain all essential information and have areas where you are able to add narrative comments.[20] These areas allow you to describe aspects of the patient's care that are not part of the standard forms. Remember to document all relevant aspects of the patient's care, including characteristics unique to some patients that might not be part of the standard forms or templates. Another problem with forms is that they are often geared toward the patient population treated most at the facility. It might be difficult to use these forms when documenting on patients with less common diagnoses.

COMPUTERIZED DOCUMENTATION

Computer-based documentation is one of the most rapidly growing areas for the use of computer technology in rehabilitation.[34] Computer-based documentation can range from basic word processing documents with fill-in form features to complex computerized documentation software packages. As with paper-based forms, initial examination/evaluations, progress notes, reevaluations, discharge summaries, and letters are common types of templates integrated into computer-based documentation packages. In some cases, documentation software is integrated with billing packages.

Benefits to computerized documentation packages include submitting information to payers electronically, building databases, tracking visits, and monitoring clinician productivity.[34] However, an important consideration of computerized documentation is the cost-benefit ratio. The benefits of using the software must offset its expense. In addition, staff training, technical support, rapid obsolescence of hardware and software, and upgrade costs are important considerations for implementing a computerized documentation system. Templates that accompany computer-based documentation packages must reflect the facility's expertise and practice or be easily modified.[34] Furthermore, the clinic must be prepared for regularly scheduled system back-ups of main and individual computer terminals so that critical information is not lost. There must also be processes for storing system back-up files. Abeln[33] suggests storing back-ups away from the computer systems themselves. Finally, there must be a mechanism to record, give reason for, and authenticate late entries.[33]

Types of computerized documentation packages include:

1. Clinicient (www.clinicient.net)
2. TurboPT (www.gssinc.com)
3. ReDoc (www.rehabdocumentation.com)
4. TalkNotes (www.provox.com) (Provox Technologies Corporation, Roanoke, Va)
5. TherAssist (www.therassist.com)
6. QuickNotes (www.qnotes.com) (Quick Notes Inc, Cooper City, Fla)

Recently, the APTA and Cedaron Medical Incorporated joined forces to create APTA Connect, a computerized documentation package that will allow scheduling, documentation, outcomes tracking, and communication with other providers.[35] For more information on APTA Connect or Cedaron Medical Incorporated you can visit the following Web sites:

1. APTA:
   http://www.apta.org/PT_Practice/For_Clinicians/aptaconnect
2. Cedaron Medical Inc:
   http://cedaron.com/cedaron/aptaconnectdata sheet 1.htm

An area of growing concern with computer-based documentation is patient confidentiality, especially when documentation software resides on a server or when health information will be transmitted electronically. The Health Insurance Portability and Accountability Act (HIPAA) provides federally regulated standards for handling individually identifiable health information during electronic transmission. HIPAA requires that facilities adopt privacy policies and procedures for maintaining secure patient records so they_ are not accessible to unauthorized personnel.[36]

REVIEW QUESTIONS

 1. List 4 types of documentation formats used in physical therapy.

2. Describe similarities and differences between narrative notes, POMRs, SOAP notes, and FOR.

3. Describe advantages and disadvantages of narrative, SOAP, POMR, and FOR documentation.

4. What type of information is found in the S, O, A, and P portions of a SOAP note?

5. When using SOAP and POMR formats, where should you place information provided by the patient's family?

6. What are positive and negative aspects of using forms and templates?

7. What are the positive and negative aspects of computerized documentation?

8. What is HIPAA? Investigate specific regulations regarding handling of individual's medical records and protected health information.

9. Do you think general computer anxiety would hinder use of computerized documentation? Why or why not? What could clinics provide to their staffs to help reduce computer anxiety when implementing computerized documentation or when training new staff?

APPLICATION EXERCISES

I.   Answer the following questions.

1. Research some of the computerized documentation packages listed in this chapter. What are some of the associated benefits of using these as indicated by the company? What is the cost? What is the policy on technical support and upgrades? Do they appear to be "user-friendly?" Why or why not?

2. Research APTA Connect. What does it offer? What are some of the advantages and disadvantages of having standardized computer software across a variety of clinics?

3. Talk to (a) clinician(s) in your area about documentation formats used at their facilities. What do they like or dislike about documentation formats currently used? What other formats have they tried? What would be the ideal documentation format?

4. Your supervising PT has asked you to work with a patient with the following problems: flaccid left upper extremity, weakness in left lower extremity, dependence with ambulation, requires assist for all transfers, unable to perform self-care or home management skills.

    *   List 3 questions that you could ask this patient when initiating a treatment session to elicit information for the subjective portion of a SOAP note.

    *   What are 3 tests, measurements, or functional activities you should document on this patient?

    *   Compare and contrast SOAP, POMR, and FOR for this patient. What would be the same in all 3? What would be different? Which of these documentation formats would be most difficult to complete for this patient?

II.   Read each statements and determine if it would belong in the S, O, A, or P portion of a SOAP note.

1. __O__   *Gait:* Ambulated 50' x 2 WBAT (R) LE c̄ min (A) x 1 and verbal cues to advance the (R) LE
2. __S__   Pt. reports that the HEP has helped improve ROM
3. __P__   Pt. will RTC 2x/wk for the next 4 wks
4. __O__   *Transfers:* bed ↔ chair c̄ mod (A) x 2
5. __A__   Pt. progressing toward goals set on the initial evaluation
6. __S__   Pt.'s wife stated that she has been assisting the pt. c̄ his HEP
7. __P__   Speak c̄ the PT about possible reeval. 2° to pt's rapid progress
8. __O__   AROM: (R) knee 0-135°
9. __A__   Improvements in knee ROM allow pt. to sit s̄ difficulty and ↑↓ stairs c̄ less difficulty *(S if pt stated)*
10. __S__   Pt. feels that he is benefiting from the strengthening exercises in that he is now able to open jars and lids (I)
11. __P__   Pt. will be seen for bid gait training
12. __S__   Pt. c/o inability to move her (L) UE and LE
13. __S__   Pt. denies use of AD PTA
14. __A__   Gait distance improved from 25' to 150' over the last week
15. __A__   Pt. demonstrating (L) neglect making her unsafe during gait and transfers
16. __O__   *Muscle Performance:* All (R) LE strength is 5/5
17. __O__   *Vitals:* HR 95 bpm, RR 12, and BP 140/95
18. __A__   Pt. has improved ability to transfer in/out of bed since initial visit
19. __P__   Will contact PT about possible d/c evaluation as pt. is no longer benefiting from the intervention
20. __A__   Pt.'s endurance is poor 2° to COPD
21. __S__   C/O inability to brush teeth and eat c̄ the (R) hand 2° ↓ AROM of the (R) elbow
22. __A__   Pt. is unable to drive or perform safe community mobility at this time
23. __A__   Edema in the (R) ankle has ↓ 2 cm.
24. __O__   Pt. dons/doffs prosthesis (I)
25. __O__   *Wound appearance:* 100% red, healthy granulation tissue c̄ minimal drainage

III.   Of the above statements, which would be considered "functional" and appropriate using FOR (Refer to p. 25 for suggestions when using FOR)?

Chapter Four

The Physical Therapy Process

Becky McKnight, PT, MS

CHAPTER OBJECTIVES

After reading this chapter, the student will be able to:

1. Describe the physical therapy process.

2. List the 5 elements of the patient/client management model.

3. Define and describe each of the 5 elements of the patient/client management model.

4. Differentiate between PT and PTA documentation responsibilities.

5. Discuss the role of documentation in the physical therapy process.

6. List types of information that can be found in an initial evaluative note.

7. Locate and use information in the initial evaluative note that will guide the selection of which data collection activities and which interventions need to be performed.

8. Locate and use information in the initial evaluative note that will assist the PTA in judging the patient's performance and outcomes and determining what course of action needs to be taken.

INTRODUCTION

It was a bright July morning. Sarah approached the outpatient physical therapy clinic with a feeling of excitement and an air of expectation. This would be her first day of patient care as a licensed physical therapist assistant. As

excited as she was, Sarah was also nervous. She knew she had an important role to play in her new position, and now she no longer had a clinical instructor or her college teachers helping her make decisions. Questions swirled through her mind as she walked in the door. "Am I really ready for this?" "Will I remember what I learned?" Her apprehension doubled as she met with John, her supervising physical therapist. As John began to discuss with Sarah the patient care activities he was directing her to perform that day her questions continued to trouble her. "Will I know what to do with the patients I will be working with?" "Will the interventions I provide be effective?" "Will John have confidence in my abilities?" Sarah's anxiety followed her throughout the morning until she sat down to review the chart for her first patient, Mrs. S.S. As she read the information about Mrs. S.S. she realized she knew exactly what to do, and she was able to approach her first patient with confidence that morning.

Sarah was able to have confidence as she began her day of patient care because she had a clear understanding of the physical therapy process. Based upon this understanding, Sarah knew what was expected of her, and she knew what to expect from John, her supervising physical therapist. Sarah's knowledge allowed her to be able to use the communication tool of the patient record to determine how she would proceed with Mrs. S.S.'s care that day.

Before you will be able to participate in the provision of physical therapy services efficiently and with confidence, as Sarah was able to do, you must start with an understanding of the entire physical therapy care process. This will enable you to appreciate the role you will play in the

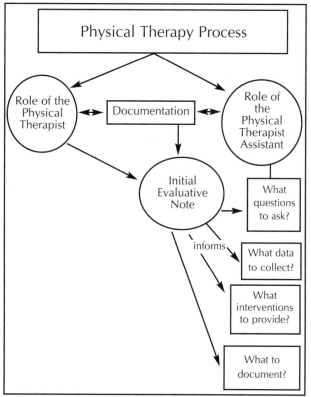

Figure 4-1. The physical therapy process and the role of documentation.

provision of physical therapy services and the role of your supervising physical therapist(s). Based upon this, you will begin to grasp how integral communication is to the entire physical therapy care process and how essential effective documentation is in ensuring patients "receive appropriate, comprehensive, efficient, and effective quality care."[7] (Figure 4-1)

THE PHYSICAL THERAPY PROCESS

The Guide to Physical Therapist Practice[7] outlines the physical therapy process through the physical therapist patient/client management model. This model describes the 5 elements necessary to ensure optimal outcomes of physical therapy services once an individual has entered into the physical therapy system. These essential components include examination, evaluation, diagnosis, prognosis, and intervention.[7] (Table 4-1)

Patient Point of Entry

Individuals enter the physical therapy system by self-referral, or they are referred to a physical therapist by another health care practitioner. Self referral, also known

as direct access, can only occur if the state practice act allows for it. Currently, 38 states have practice acts that allow for some degree of direct access.[37] Individuals in these states can legally seek physical therapy services when they feel they have a need for physical therapy without first obtaining a physician's order. Alternatively, patients can enter the physical therapy system when they are referred by another health care provider. Common referral sources include physicians, chiropractors, and dentists. A patient's initial introduction to physical therapy is often after hospitalization for disease or injury. At other times individuals will enter into the system through outpatient services, home health services, or school-based services.

The Patient/Client Management Model

Once an individual has entered the physical therapy system, the physical therapist will initiate care through the examination process. The examination process is composed of 3 components: history-taking, systems review, and tests and measures. During the history-taking portion of the examination, the physical therapist will gather various pieces of information from the medical record, or from the patient, that will help put into context the reason the individual is seeking physical therapy services. Types of data gathered during this process include:

- General demographics (age, sex, race, etc)
- Social history
- Employment/work (job/school/play)
- Growth and development
- Living environment
- General health status
- Social/health habits (past and current)
- Family history
- Current condition(s)/chief complaint(s)
- Functional status and activity level
- Medications
- Other clinical tests (lab tests, radiology reports)[7]

After obtaining a picture of the patient's condition and concerns, the physical therapist will perform a systems review. During a systems review, the physical therapist assesses the patient's overall medical health by reviewing the cardiovascular/pulmonary system, the integumentary system, the musculoskeletal system, the neuromuscular system, cognitive skills, and communication abilities. Based upon information gathered during this process the physical therapist will select and perform appropriate tests and measures.[7] Test and measures are methods and techniques the therapist uses to gather data needed to determine the diagnosis and the intervention strategy. Tests and measures are also used to evaluate outcomes and to note the patient's progress.

Table 4-1

THE FIVE ELEMENTS OF THE PATIENT/CLIENT MANAGEMENT MODEL

Element	Who/When	Includes	Source of Information	Purpose
1. Examination	Performed by the PT on all patients prior to the intervention	a.) History	Chart Review Patient Interview	Aids the PT in determining the most appropriate plan of care
		b.) Systems Review	Examination of various body systems including: Cardiovascular System, Integumentary System, Musculoskeletal System, Neuromuscular System, Communication, Cognition, Language, etc	
		c.) Tests and Measurements	Range of motion measurements, gross muscle testing, sensation testing, girth, etc	
2. Evaluation	After the Examination, the PT makes a clinical judgment based on findings			Allows others (including the PTA) insight to the anticipated level of improvement, intervention plan, and frequency and duration of services
3. Diagnosis	PT assigns a Physical Therapy Diagnosis			
4. Prognosis (Includes the Plan of Care)	PT determines the predicted level of improvement, treatment goals, expected outcomes, duration and frequency of treatment, and interventions to be used			
5. Intervention	Done by the PT or PTA to produce changes in the patient's condition	a.) Coordination, Communication, and Documentation	Working with other disciplines including physicians, occupational therapists, nurses, etc	Establish and maintain an open line of communication between disciplines
		b.) Patient/Client-related instructions	Includes communicating with the patient and family	Informing patients and families
		c.) Procedural Interventions	Includes things like hot packs, cold packs, range of motion exercises, strengthening exercise, gait training, transfer training, etc	Decrease inflammation, decrease pain, increase motion, etc

The physical therapist evaluates the information gathered during the examination process and makes clinical judgments about the findings to determine a physical therapy diagnosis and prognosis and to establish the plan of care. This clinical decision-making process is known as the evaluation process.

The physical therapy plan of care is developed in collaboration with the patient and is based on the examination, evaluation, diagnosis, and prognosis. The plan of care includes goals and anticipated outcomes, the expected frequency and duration of services, and at least a general statement of interventions to be used.[38] Every physical therapy plan of care must include succinct, "measurable and time limited"[7] goals. Goals serve as the tool to which outcomes are compared. This allows for assessment of the effectiveness of the plan of care and assessment of the patient's progress. A well written plan of care will delineate the interventions, treatment parameters, purpose of the interventions, progression parameters, and, if indicated, precautions.

Once the plan of care has been established, direct intervention can begin. A properly constructed physical therapy plan of care will incorporate appropriate interventions to ensure optimal outcomes and should include the following 3 components: (1) coordination, communication, and documentation; (2) patient-related instruction; and (3) procedural interventions.[1] Historically, when discussing a physical therapy plan of care, the emphasis was on the physical agents or therapeutic activities that would be utilized. This correlates with the third component (procedural interventions) of a properly constructed physical therapy plan of care. More recently, there has been a growing appreciation for, and a shift toward recognizing the importance of, the other 2 components (coordination, communication, and documentation *and* patient/client-related instructions) of the physical therapy process. The patient/client management model now formalizes their inclusion into the plan of care.

As the physical therapy interventions are initiated, the patient's progress toward the established goals (outcomes) is monitored. At various times within the process, reexamination may occur to formally document the patient's status and progress, or lack thereof. Based upon the findings from the reexamination, the physical therapist may alter the plan of care.

As part of the plan of care, the physical therapist will develop discharge plans. Depending upon a variety of variables (the environment, the established goals, the patient's progress, and the prognosis), the discharge plan may be to transfer to another therapy service in another environment (acute rehab, skilled nursing, outpatient, or home health). When established goals are met, discharge from an episode of care occurs. Additionally, discontinuation of physical therapy services may occur without established goals being achieved. When this happens the physical therapist should document the reason the established goals were not met.[7] Upon discharge or discontinuation, the patient/client may be given a home exercise program or may be placed on a maintenance therapy program to try to maintain maximum functional capabilities in the absence of skilled therapeutic intervention. The establishment of a home exercise program, whether during the episode of physical therapy care or at the conclusion of physical therapy services, should be a part of the plan of care established by the physical therapist.

PHYSICAL THERAPIST AND PHYSICAL THERAPIST ASSISTANT ROLES

APTA's *Direction and Supervision of the Physical Therapist Assistant*[39] clearly outlines the roles the physical therapist and the physical therapist assistant play within the patient/client management model. The physical therapist is the recognized professional who establishes, guides, and directs all aspects of the provision of physical therapy services. It is the responsibility of the physical therapist to interpret referrals; perform the initial examination and evaluation; establish the physical therapy diagnosis, prognosis, and plan of care (including goals and a discharge plan); and determine which interventions require the clinical decision-making skill of a physical therapist and which interventions can be provided by a physical therapist assistant. In addition, the physical therapist is responsible for reexamination of the patient and revision of the plan of care when indicated. The physical therapist is also directly responsible for ensuring appropriate documentation for all physical therapy services.

As a physical therapist assistant, your role in patient care activities will be within the intervention portion of the patient/client management model. You will implement selected interventions of the plan of care as directed by the physical therapist. You will play an integral role with all 3 aspects of the intervention and should be prepared to participate in coordination, communication, and documentation; patient-related instruction; and procedural interventions. You must be able to utilize clinical judgments regarding the patient's response(s) to the intervention being providing and determine when to consult with the physical therapist about the patient's progress. At times, you will need to assist with data collection to provide information useful in determining the patient's progress toward the established goals. As a physical therapist assistant, you will be able to modify details of the treatment program, within the established plan of care as directed by the supervising physical therapist, to ensure the greatest efficiency and effectiveness of the interventions being provided (Figure 4-2).[38-40]

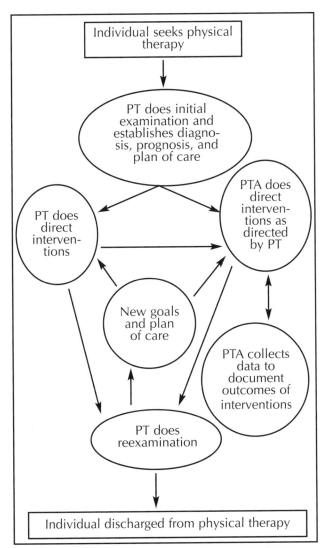

Figure 4-2. The physical therapy process. Adapted from *Introduction to Physical Therapy*. 2nd ed, Pagliarulo, Pathways of delegation (decision tree) involving the physical therapist (PT) and physical therapist assistant (PTA), pg 56, 2001, with permission from Elsevier.

Whether it is provided by the therapist directly or by an assistant, the physical therapist is responsible for all aspects of the physical therapy service being provided at all times. As a physical therapist assistant you will only be responsible for providing the patient care interventions that are delegated to you by your supervising physical therapist. You will share the responsibility with the physical therapist for guaranteeing that you only provide patient care interventions within your education and skill level and within legal parameters for the state in which you practice.[40,41] It will also be your responsibility to clearly and accurately document all patient care activities that you provide.

For the provision of physical therapy services to be efficient and effective, a positive working relationship must exist between the physical therapist and the assistant. This type of relationship is characterized by trust and mutual respect, as well as an appreciation for individual differences. A hallmark of a good working relationship is excellent communication.[40]

COORDINATION, COMMUNICATION, AND DOCUMENTATION

To ensure optimal outcomes from physical therapy services, it is imperative that appropriate coordination of services and communication related to those services occurs. Both of these components can be facilitated through, and should (at a minimum) be outlined in, concise documentation. Collaboration of services includes working with a variety of health care providers and, most importantly, the patient and the patient's family/support structure. Collaboration only occurs in the presence of rich communication. To be able to function within the health care delivery system you will need to effectively communicate with other members of the health care delivery team. Effective communication includes appropriate verbal and nonverbal communication as well as accurate documentation.[40] Documentation will provide the foundation upon which all clinical activity occurs.

UTILIZING THE PHYSICAL THERAPY DOCUMENTATION

APTA's *Guidelines for Physical Therapy Documentation*[7] advises documentation of physical therapy services occur at the following times: (1) at the initiation of services (the initial evaluation), (2) to detail all interventions provided, (3) to describe the patient's status and progress, (4) for all reexaminations or reevaluations, and (5) at the end of the episode of physical therapy care. Documentation regarding physical therapy services begins with the physical therapist's initial evaluative note. The initial evaluative note will provide a clear picture of the patient by including pertinent history, risk factors, and results of tests and measures. The evaluative note will document the physical therapist's professional judgment about the patient's condition including the physical therapy diagnosis, prognosis, and anticipated goals. Finally, the evaluative note will include recommendations and a treatment plan.[7]

As a PTA you will use the physical therapy initial evaluative note as a reference for each patient contact. The initial evaluative note should provide the framework upon which all patient-related activities you engage in are based. From the initial evaluative note, you should be able to obtain a clear picture of what is happening with the patient and how physical therapy services will be administered to address the patient's problems. You will have at least a general idea of what to anticipate when you work with the patient.

Table 4-2

WHERE THE ELEMENTS OF THE PATIENT/CLIENT MANAGEMENT MODEL CAN BE FOUND IN A SOAP NOTE

Element of Patient/Client Management Model — *SOAP Initial Evaluative Note*

Element of Patient/Client Management Model	SOAP Initial Evaluative Note
Examination — History —	Problem
	Subjective (when taken from the patient)
	Objective (when taken from the medical record)
Systems Review	Objective
Tests and Measures	Objective
Evaluation	Assessment
Diagnosis	Assessment
Prognosis	Assessment
Intervention	Plan

SOAP Initial Evaluative Note

Let's look at what a typical physical therapy evaluative note written in the SOAP format looks like and discuss how you can utilize this information to determine what you will do with the patient. In the evaluative note you will find information related to the examination process in the problem, subjective, and objective sections of the note. Information about the evaluative process, as well as the diagnosis and prognosis, can be found in the assessment portion of the note. Finally, the intervention program will be documented primarily within the plan section (Table 4-2). We will look at each section individually, and then we will discuss how you will utilize the information to make decisions about what to do for patient care.

Problem (Pr)

The Problem section of a SOAP note is the first part of the initial evaluative note and provides information about the patient's reason for seeking physical therapy services. The problem can be derived from the history-taking portion of the examination, from the physician's referral, or from the medical record. The following information *may* be found in this section:

- Patient's chief complaint
- Medical diagnosis
- Physical therapy diagnosis
- Functional limitations

Box 4-1

Example of Entry Information in Problem Section of a Evaluative Note

Outpatient Physical Therapy Evaluation

Patient: S.S.
Age: 53 y/o
Date of Eval: 11/14/02
Referral: PT to eval & tx
Referring Physician: Dr. Mark Long

Pr: Progressive Remitting type MS with balance and coordination deficits

---

- Information gleaned from the medical record, such as:
  - Recent or past surgeries
  - Past conditions or diseases
  - Present conditions or diseases
  - Results of medical tests (Box 4-1)

In many settings, the problem section only includes the medical diagnosis and/or referral information with the remainder listed elsewhere.

Box 4-2

Example of Information in the Subjective Section of an Evaluative Note

S: *Current Condition:* This 53 y/o female reports she was diagnosed with progressive MS 2 years ago. On 11/4/03 she had an exacerbation of her MS that lead her to be hospitalized for 3 days of IV anti-inflammatory medications. She was d/c'd to home on 11/7/03 with a wheeled walker. She was receiving PT while in the hospital. During her follow up visit with her physician on 11/11/02 the pt. requested more PT due to balance and coordination problems. The pt. currently c/o "being unsteady on my feet," and being "clumsy with everything." Pt. reports she will be receiving OT to address coordination problems that interfere with daily functioning.

Living Environment: The pt. lives at home with her husband and 17 y/o son. Three steps with a railing to enter her one level home.

Functional Status: Pt. states she was previously (I) with all ADL's and gait without an assistive device. Pt.'s husband works during the day and her son goes to school. Her husband has been taking time off from work to stay with her during the day but will have to return to work this week. The pt. has various friends and family who have agreed to help her during the day until she is safe to be alone at home.

Employment Status: She is normally employed as a bank teller but is unable to return to work at this time due to fatigue issues and "clumsiness."

Patient's Goals: The patient states she would like to be able to walk without an assistive device, to return to work, and to be able to do housework.

Box 4-3

Example of Information in the Objective Section of an Evaluative Note

O: Systems Review:
Cardiovascular/Pulmonary System: Unimpaired. BP: 130/85. HR: 88 bpm. RR: 20
Integumentary System: Unimpaired.
Musculoskeletal System: Gross symmetry unimpaired. Gross ROM unimpaired. Gross strength impaired equally bilaterally UEs & LEs.
Neuromuscular System: Mobility impaired. Motor function impaired. Balance impaired.
Communication: Unimpaired.
Cognition: Unimpaired.

Tests & Measures & Observation:
Sensation: Pt. displays sharp/dull, proprioception & kinesthesia to (B) LE's from knees down.
MMT: 4-/5 to 4+/5 throughout all 4 extremities utilizing standard test positions.
Mobility: (I) with bed mobility, supine ↔ sit and sit ↔ stand requires SBA for safety due to ataxia. Pt. ambulates 200' with wheeled walker and min (A) on level surfaces, demonstrating truncal & (B) LE ataxia.
Balance: Sitting static good-, dynamic fair+, standing static fair, dynamic fair-
Coordination: Pt. displays ataxia of all 4 extremities during functional tasks and during coordination tests including finger-nose-finger and heel-shin tests.
Endurance: Fair for the above activities. Pt. fatigues after 15 minutes of activities.

Subjective (S)

The subjective section of a SOAP note provides all pertinent data that is obtained from the patient or the patient's family or caregiver. The subjective information is also a component of the history-taking portion of the examination. The following information can be found in this section:

- Patient's current and past medical history
- Patient's symptoms or complaints
- Factors that cause the symptoms or complaints
- Patient's prior level of function
- Patient's lifestyle/occupation/societal roles
- Patient's goals (Box 4-2)

Objective (O)

The objective section of a SOAP note includes information related to tests or interventions which can be reproduced. Objective data is a component of the examination. The following types of information can be found in the objective section:

- Information gathered through:
  - Tests and Measures
  - Observation
- Interventions provided
- Patient's response to interventions provided
- Patient's education (Box 4-3)

Assessment (A)

The assessment section of a SOAP note provides the physical therapist's evaluation. In this section, the physical therapist will summarize the "S" and "O" information and

---

Box 4-4

Example of Information in the Assessment Section of an Evaluative Note

A: Pt.'s motor deficits including balance, coordination, and strength deficits prevent her from mobilizing independently. The patient is unable to maintain her current employment and is not able to meet her roles as a wife and mother. The patient's rehab potential may be limited due to diagnosis of progressive remitting type MS. The patient's fatigue level will limit her participation but with continued efforts the patient maybe able to achieve her stated goals. Will provide a 2 week trial of physical therapy intervention to determine the patient's potential.

STG's: To be achieved after 2 weeks of physical therapy:

1. (I) & safe c̄ all transfers including sup ↔ sit & sit ↔ stand to allow patient greater (I) at home.
2. Pt. will ambulate with wheeled walker and SBA for safety on level surfaces and with CGA on uneven surfaces and stairs.
3. Increase general endurance so pt. can tolerate 30 minutes of functional and therapeutic activities to meet the above functional goals.
4. Increase strength ½ grade throughout all extremities to meet the above functional goals.
5. Improve coordination of extremities to meet the above functional goals.
6. Increase balance: static & dynamic sitting to good, static standing fair+ to meet the above functional goals.

LTG's: No LTG's set at this time until potential has been assessed over the next 2 weeks of therapy intervention.

Box 4-5

Example of Information in the Plan Section of an Evaluative Note

P: Will be seen 3x/wk as an outpatient. Pt. will receive strengthening exercises, balance & coordination activities, functional mobility training, and gait training. Will continue gait training with wheeled walker until (I) gait with wheeled walker is achieved then will progress to gait training with other (A) device as indicated.

John Jordon, PT

- Explanation of any difficulties with obtaining S or O data
- Suggestions for further testing, treatment, or referrals (Box 4-4)

Plan (P)

The plan section of a SOAP note provides the written plan for physical therapy services and is part of the established plan of care. The following types of information may be found in the plan section:

- Plan for intervention activities to occur
  - Collaboration/communication
  - Pt. related education
  - Procedural interventions
- Frequency and duration of therapy services
- Treatment progression
- Plans for further assessment or reassessment
- Equipment needs
- Referral to other services (Box 4-5)

How to Use the Initial Evaluative Note

When you review the initial evaluative note you will want to glean specific information from each section to assist you in determining what you need to do. The problem section will provide you with the patient's diagnosis. You will immediately be able to get a general idea of what to expect from the patient. For example, in the patient case above, as soon as Sarah read that S.S. has a diagnosis of progressive remitting MS, she had a general idea of what to expect from the patient based upon her knowledge of that disease process. Further information provided in the remainder of the note helped Sarah to fill in the details so she had a clearer picture of what to expect of S.S.'s status and performance.

begin to outline the plan of care. The following will be found in the assessment section:

- Physical therapist's interpretation of S and O data
- Goals
- Identification of impairments and functional limitations
- Physical therapy diagnosis
- Prognosis/rehabilitation potential
- Justification for goals/treatment plan

As you review the subjective information you will want to think about what questions you might want to ask the patient. In S.S.'s case, Sarah may want to ask how the assistance from friends and family has been working out. You also want to think about other pieces of information you want to be listening for as you provide your intervention. Frequently, patients share important information days or weeks after the initial evaluation. This information can be useful in providing a more efficient plan of care. For example, if S.S. were to share a history of a previous (R) arthroscopic knee surgery with occasional knee pain, Sarah would want to document this information in the patient's chart and communicate it to the supervising physical therapist. This may help to explain discrepancies in strength gains between the LEs if any are noticed in future sessions.

When you review the objective information, you want to picture in your mind how the patient will look and act. This will allow you to anticipate appropriate responses to therapeutic intervention and will help you identify inappropriate responses. As Sarah works with S.S., she will expect the patient to fatigue and will build rest breaks into the therapy session depending upon the level of activities performed. However, Sarah will not expect any specific complaints of pain. If S.S. begins complaining of localized pain in her (L) ankle, Sarah would know to consult with the physical therapist. Also, as you review the objective data, you will want to decide what data collection activities you need to perform to determine the patient's response to the therapeutic intervention. To monitor S.S.'s progress toward the established goals and responses to the interventions provided, Sarah will observe S.S.'s functional mobility status and then will perform MMT and balance and coordination assessments.

As you read the assessment portion of the note, you will be able to outline in your mind how the patient should progress. This will guide you in the day-to-day decisions about what needs to happen with the patient. Review of the plan section will tell you the amount of time to work with the patient and will inform you what activities you should perform and what resources you should use. Based upon John's assessment of S.S., Sarah would not be alarmed if the patient did not show significant improvements over the course of the treatment plan.

Questions to Ask

To assist you in preparing for patient interaction when you review an initial evaluative note, or any subsequent intervention/progress note, you will want to ask a series of questions. The following are example questions that will guide you in determining what you need to do.

- "What do I need to know to be able to effectively treat this patient?" Information that you will want to look for includes the medical diagnosis; the physical therapy diagnosis; any listed precautions, contraindications, impairments, functional limitations, or disabilities; established goals; and the treatment plan.

- "What do I know about this diagnosis that will impact how I provide the intervention?" Eg, a diagnosis of Guillian Barré would indicate that you would not be aggressive with therapeutic exercise.

- "What other diagnosis does this patient have that might impact performance in physical therapy?" Eg, a patient recovering from a hip fracture that underwent an ORIF and must follow restricted weight bearing precautions may also have a diagnosis of Alzheimer's disease. Due to the cognitive dysfunction, this patient will have difficulty maintaining the correct weight bearing.

- "Is there any other information I need that is not found in the evaluative note?" If the answer is yes, you will want to seek out the information from the appropriate source (may or may not be the physical therapist). Eg, you know that a routine Doppler was performed after a total knee replacement. You will want to check with the nurse to make sure the Doppler came back clear before proceeding with the therapy session.

- "What questions do I need to be prepared to ask the patient?" Eg, if the evaluative note indicates the patient reported being in pain, you will want to ask the patient about his/her pain level.

- "What data do I need to collect to help demonstrate the patient's response to the treatment plan?" Eg, monitoring blood pressure with a patient who is status post coronary artery bypass graft surgery.

- "What equipment do I need to provide the intervention?" Eg, gait belt, walker, ultrasound machine.

- "What type of responses might cause me to decide not to initiate treatment or to stop treatment once it has started?" Eg, you enter the room to work with a patient who is recovering from back surgery. The patient indicates he has been having strong pain in his left calf all morning long. You would know not to initiate therapy until you consulted with the nurse and the physical therapist regarding this new complaint.

- "What information needs to be included in my treatment/progress note?" You do not need to include information in the progress note that was found to be within normal parameters in the evaluative note. Eg, if the evaluative note indicated the patient had no cognitive or communication deficits, you do not need to repeat that in your progress note as long as there is not a change in that status.

REVIEW QUESTIONS

1. Define and describe the 5 elements of the patient/client management model.

2. Next to each component of the patient/client management model indicate if the PT, the PTA, or both participate(s) in that process.

        _____Examination
        _____Evaluation
        _____Diagnosis
        _____Prognosis
        _____Intervention

3. For each of the following components of the patient/client management model indicate where this information can be found within an initial evaluative note written in the SOAP note format. Write Pr for problem, S for subjective, O for objective, A for assessment, and P for plan.

        _____Prognosis
        _____Examination: History-Taking
        _____Evaluation
        _____Intervention
        _____Examination: Systems Review
        _____Diagnosis
        _____Examination: Tests & Measures

4. For each of the following types of information that may be found in a physical therapy evaluative note indicate where the information would be documented in the SOAP note format. Write Pr for problem, S for subjective, O for objective, A for assessment, and P for plan.

        _____Rehabilitation potential
        _____Patient education provided
        _____Medical diagnosis
        _____Patient's complaints
        _____Equipment needed
        _____Goals
        _____Recent surgeries
        _____Patient's prior level of function
        _____Interventions provided
        _____Results of tests

5. Discuss the importance of documentation and communication within the intervention provided in the patient/client management model.

APPLICATION EXERCISES

I. Reference the physical therapy practice act for your state of residence for language regarding direct access. Does your state allow for direct access? Are there any restrictions or provisions related to direct access in the practice act?

II. Using the following case examples (Box 4-6 through Box 4-8), practice reviewing initial evaluative notes to prepare for a treatment session. Use the following guiding questions to work through this process.
- "What do I need to know to be able to effectively treat this patient?"
- "What do I know about this diagnosis that will impact how I provide the intervention?"
- "What other diagnoses does this patient have that might impact performance in physical therapy?"
- "Is there any other information I need that is not found in the evaluative note?"
- "What questions do I need to be prepared to ask the patient?"
- "What data do I need to collect to help demonstrate the patient's response to the treatment plan?"
- "What equipment do I need to provide for the intervention?"
- "What type of responses might cause me to decide not to initiate treatment or to stop treatment once it has started?"
- "What information needs to be included in my treatment/progress note?"

Box 4-6

Evaluative Note for a Patient Who Underwent a THA

Anytown Community Hospital
Skilled Nursing Facility

Physical Therapy Evaluation

Patient: J.M.
Age: 76 y/o
Date: 04/04/05
Referral: Physical therapy for gait and strengthening. Anterior hip precautions, WBAT
Referring Physician: Dr. Mark John

Pr: (L) THA 03/30/05. HTN; two previous TIA's approx. 1 year ago.

S: *Complaint:* The patient states he does have some soreness but in general his hip pain is less than before the surgery; rates pain as 1-2/10 and states it hurts worse at the end of the day.

Living Environment/Social Support: The patient reports he lives at home with his wife. His wife is generally in good health and is active in the community but pt. is concerned about being a "burden" on his wife when he returns home. Pt. states he has 3 steps with railing on one side to enter his one level home.

Prior Level of Function/Activities: The patient states he was previously (I) with ADL's and gait without (A) device; his hobbies include yard work and doing crossword puzzles; he is retired; pt. normally attended church twice a week and met with friends for coffee 3-4 times a week; pt. enjoys fly fishing 3-4 times a month "depending upon the weather."

Patient Goals: The patient states he would like to return to his previous level of activity and specifically is hoping to participate in a fishing tournament this fall.

O: **Systems Review:**

Cardiovascular/Pulmonary System: Unimpaired. BP: 130/85. HR: 88 bpm. RR: 20

Integumentary System: Healing scar (L) Hip, staples intact, no drainage noted.

Musculoskeletal System: Gross strength general decrease (B) UE's and (R) LE; (L) LE impaired due to recent surgery. Gross ROM (L) LE restricted due to orthopedic precautions; other extremities and trunk unimpaired.

Neuromuscular System: Balance & motor control unimpaired. Functional mobility impaired.

Communication: Unimpaired.

Cognition: Unimpaired.

Tests & Measures & Observation:

Strength: 4/5 to 4+/5 throughout (B) UE's and (R) LE. (L) hip musculature not tested at this time due to recent surgery. Appears 2/5 with functional mobility. (L) knee strength 3+/5, ankle strength 5/5.

Mobility: Scooting in bed min (A) to assist (L) LE. Supine ↔ sit with Mod (A), Sit ↔ Stand with min (A).

Gait: Pt. ambulated 50' with walker and min (A) WBAT (L) LE. Pt. needed frequent v/c's for proper walker placement 2° tendency to place walker too far in front of him.

Treatment: Initiated bed mobility training, transfer training, and gait training using front wheeled walker; AAROM to (L) LE, including ankle pumps, quad sets, ham sets, glut sets, SAQ, SLR, hip abd and heel slides 2 x 10. Pt. required min (A) with SAQs and heel slides and mod (A) with SLRs and hip abd.

Pt. Education: Pt. was instructed in hip precautions. Pt. was able to repeat hip precautions after 10 minutes of alternate activities.

continued

Patient: J.M.

A: Pt's decreased strength (L) LE is limiting his functional (I). Pt. is unable to return home at this time due to dependence with mobility and need to learn hip precautions to protect recent THA surgery. This pt. is very motivated and does not have significant co-morbidities and therefore has excellent rehab potential.

Problem List:

1. Decreased strength (L) LE
2. Dependent mobility
3. Dependent gait
4. Does not know hip precautions for functional tasks

STGs: To be met within 2 days

1. Pt. will require SBA-CGA with all bed mobility & transfers.
2. Pt. will ambulate 100' with walker & CGA on level surfaces.
3. Increase (L) LE strength to 3/5 throughout hip and 4-/5 knee to be able to meet the above functional goals.
4. Pt. will be able to verbalize all hip precautions and will demonstrate understanding of precautions during basic transfers and gait activities.

LTGs: To be met within 7 days to allow the patient to return home with his wife.

1. Pt. will be (I) with all bed mobility & transfers and car transfers with min (A) of wife.
2. Pt. will ambulate 200' with walker (I) on level surface & up and down 3 steps utilizing railing on one side with SBA of wife.
3. Increase (L) LE strength to 3+/5 throughout hip and 4/5 knee to be able to meet the above functional goals.
4. Pt. will display good understanding of hip precautions during all functional activities including car transfers and gait on stairs.

P: PT BID, for ROM/strengthening exercises, transfer training including car transfers, gait training including gait on stairs, and education regarding hip precautions with all functional tasks.

Ted Orlando, PT

Box 4-7

Evaluative Note for a Patient Recovering from a Brainstem CVA

Anytown Community Hospital
Subacute Rehabilitation

Physical Therapy Evaluation

Patient: D.W.
Age: 68 y/o
Date: 05/26/04
Referral: Physical therapy to evaluate and treat as advised
Referring Physician: Dr. Sue Morton

Pr: Brainstem CVA 05/21/04; Type 2 diabetes; (R) carotid endarterectomy 07/02, and 3 previous TIA's.

S: *Current Condition*: Pt. reports that on 05/21/04 she awoke to find she could not get herself out of bed. She had been experiencing feelings of fatigue and weakness the evening before and had gone to bed early. Pt.'s husband called emergency services and she was transported to the hospital where the diagnosis of brainstem CVA was made.

Patient Complaint: The patient c/o weakness on the (R) side of her body and "clumsiness" with her (L) arm. She states she is unable to anything on her own at this point. The pt. admits to being very frustrated and just "wants to give up."

continued

Patient: D.W.

Living Environment/Social Support: Pt. reports she previously lived at home with her husband in a one-story ranch style home with 1 step to enter. The pt. and her husband have three children. One son lives in the area and can be available to assist some. The other two children do not live in the area. Her husband owns his own business as an electrician and will be able to cut back his "hours of work" to help her if needed.

Prior Level of Function/Activities: Pt. states she has always been a "housewife" and is sure her husband would be unable to "run the home". Pt's social activities include being involved in a reading club that meets monthly and going to church weekly. Pt. also reports she occasionally keeps her neighbor's children in the evenings. The children are 5 and 8 years old.

Patient's Goals: She states she and her husband are hoping that she can eventually return home. She would like to return to as many of her previous activities as possible but voices she understands she may need to use a cane, walker, or wheelchair to get around. Pt. is most concerned about being able to take care of her home including doing dishes, laundry, and general house cleaning tasks.

O: **Systems Review**:

Cardiovascular/Pulmonary System: BP: 128/70. HR: 74 bpm. RR: 20

Integumentary System: Unimpaired.

Musculoskeletal System: Gross ROM unimpaired. Gross strength impaired throughout trunk and (B) UE's & LE's (R) > (L).

Neuromuscular System: Balance & motor control impaired throughout trunk and all four extremities. Functional mobility impaired for all tasks.

Communication: Mild slurred speech. Pt. easily understood.

Cognition: Unimpaired.

Other: Urinary catheter noted.

Tests & Measures & Observation:

Observation: Pt. grossly obese.

Sensory: Pt. demonstrates normal light & gross touch, pain/thermal and diminished proprioception/kinesthesia on (L) and mildly diminished light & gross touch, pain/thermal, and proprioception/kinesthesia on (R) throughout trunk and extremities.

Tone: The patient displayed mild hypotonia (R) UE & LE and normal tone (L) UE & LE.

MMT:	(R)	(L)
Shoulder:		
Flexors	2/5	4/5
Extensors	1/5	4/5
Abductors	1/5	4/5
Adductors	2/5	5/5
Medial Rotators	2/5	5/5
Lateral Rotators	1/5	4-/5
Elbow:		
Flexors	2/5	5/5
Extensors	0/5	4+/5
Wrist:		
Flexors	1/5	4/5
Extensors	0/5	4-/5
Grip:	5#	28#
Hip:		
Flexors	1/5	4-/5
Extensors	3/5	4-/5
Abductors	0/5	4-/5
Adductors	3+/5	5/5

continued

Patient: D.W.

Knee:

Flexors	0/5	4/5
Extensors	2+/5	5/5

Ankle:

Dorsiflexors	0/5	4+/5
Plantarflexors	1/5	5/5

Balance: Sitting static fair-, dynamic poor; Standing not assessed at this time.

Coordination: Unable to assess (R) side due to weakness. (L) UE & LE demonstrates diminished coordination with all activities. Note apraxia and pass pointing during exercises.

Bed Mobility: Max (A) with rolling and scooting in bed.

Transfers: Max (A) supine ↔ sit. Unable to perform sit ↔ stand at this time. Bed ↔ mat or bed at this time is via Hoyer due to patient's large size, poor balance, and weakness.

A: This obese pt. has very severe functional disabilities. Pt. is motivated and pleasant to work with. Due to the severe deficits prognosis for significant recovery is poor however the pt. and her husband want to try to get the pt. back home. A trial of structured aggressive therapy is indicated to see how much functional return is possible for this pt. and to educate her husband on how to provide any necessary care.

Problem List:

1. Decreased strength (R) > (L).
2. Decreased coordination (L) UE & LE.
3. Decreased balance.
4. Dependent with all mobility.

STGs: Within 2 weeks the pt. will display:

1. Mod (A) for bed mobility and supine ↔ sit.
2. Max (A) for bed ↔ w/c slideboard transfer.
3. Fair static and Fair- dynamic sitting balance.
4. Increase strength ½ grade throughout to be able to achieve functional goals.
5. Improve coordination (L) UE & LE to be able to achieve functional goals.

LTGs: Within 4 weeks the pt. will display:

1. Min (A) for bed mobility and supine ↔ sit.
2. Mod (A) for bed ↔ w/c slideboard transfer.
3. Fair+ static and Fair dynamic sitting balance.
4. Increase strength 1 grade throughout to be able to achieve functional goals.
5. Improve coordination (L) UE & LE to be able to achieve functional goals.

Pt.'s husband will:

1. Safely assist pt. with bed mobility and all transfers.

P: PT BID for neuromuscular reeducation, strengthening exercises, endurance activities, mobility training, and family education. Will assess pt's equipment needs for home use and facility acquisition of the equipment. Pt. will require at minimum a wheelchair and a BSC. Prior to discharge recommend pt. & pt's husband stay in the independence apartment to assess their ability to manage in a "home-like" environment. Anticipate continued therapy through home health services will be needed. If patient demonstrates good recovery over her rehab stay may recommend an extension of her stay to work toward greater independence.

Joe Jackson, PT

Box 4-8

Evaluative Note for a Patient who Suffered from an Elbow Fracture

Anytown Community Hospital
Outpatient Rehabilitation Services

Physical Therapy Evaluation

Patient: B.H.
Age: 85 y/o
Date: 09/26/05
Referral: PT for ROM and strengthening to the (L) elbow.
Referring Physician: Dr. Jeff Gordon

Pr: (L) Elbow fracture s/p ORIF 8/18/05; (L) hip fx s/p ORIF 1/05

S: *Current Condition:* Pt. states she broke her arm when she missed a step coming out of her house into her garage 08/18/05; pt.'s husband took her to the emergency room; she had surgery the same day and returned home the next day. During a follow up visit to the doctor on 09/21/05 the cast was removed. Pt. states she is coming to PT to get her "arm working again."

Patient Complaint: Pt. reports her (L) UE seems to ache all the time especially over the weekend since her cast was removed. Pt. ranks her pain as 2/10 at rest, 3-4/10 with activities, 6-7/10 during stretching/ROM exercises. Pt.reports she still is occasionally using painkillers prescribed by the physician and reports relief of her pain with meds.

Living Environment/Social Support: Pt. lives at home with spouse. Denies any steps to negotiate. Pt. reports prior to accident she was (I) with ADL's and gait without (A) device. Pt. does own walker from previous (L) LE surgery; pt. report she has needed assistance with self-care and ADL's such as bathing and dressing due to pain and stiffness since her surgery. Pt. & spouse both retired. Pt. states she likes to garden.

Patient Goals: Pt. states she wants to return to her normal function.

O: *Palpation:* There is generalized soreness upon palpation of the entire (L) elbow region. Pt. also displays tenderness in the (L) brachioradialis muscle.

Inspection: The pt. displays a well healed incision on the elbow.

ROM: (B) Shoulder AROM WNL's throughout

		(R)	(L)
PROM:	Elbow extension/flexion	0° to 150°	90° to 130°
	Forearm supination	0° to 90°	0° to 45°
	Forearm pronation	0° to 90°	0° to 35°
	Wrist flexion	0° to 75°	0°
	Wrist extension	0° to 80°	0° to 45°

The patient is unable to make a complete fist with the (L) hand due to discomfort and "stiffness." Formal measurements of finger joints not performed this date due to patient needing to get to a personal function. To be deferred to next session.

Strength: (R) UE 4+/5 - 5/5 throughout all musculature. (L) shoulder 4-/5, (L) elbow pt. unable to tolerate any resistance does perform against gravity showing 3/5 of biceps and triceps. Grip strength (R) 40#, (L) 25#.

Intervention: Patient received MHP x 20 mins to (L) elbow and (L) hand. Gentle stretching and mobilization to elbow joints followed this. PT performed AAROM to (L) elbow, wrist, and hand 10 repetitions.

continued

Patient: B.H.

Patient Education: The patient was instructed in gentle self ROM techniques. Pt. was issued a written HEP of these ROM activities (see copy in pt. chart). Pt. was advised to use prescription pain medication approximately 30 minutes before the next therapy session to increase tolerance to the activities.

A: The patient displays limited ROM, decreased strength, and (L) hand edema which are impeding her functional tasks at home. The patient had an increase in pain to 6-7/10 during therapeutic ROM and stretching.

Short Term Goals: To be achieved within 5 treatment sessions. All impairment goals listed are to facilitate the pt. to be able to be (I) with self-care activities.

(1.) Decrease edema in the (L) hand.

(2.) Increase (L) wrist ROM to WNL's.

(3.) Increase elbow flexion to 0° to 140° and extension to 140° to 0°

Long Term Goals: To be achieved within 14 treatment sessions. All impairment goals listed are to facilitate pt. to be able to return to normal activities including house work and gardening.

(1.) Increase strength in the (L) elbow and hand to 4/5-4+/5 throughout.

(2.) Increase (L) elbow ROM to WNL's

(3.) The patient will be (I) with basic ADL's and IADL's.

P: Patient to receive PT 3x/week for modalities, ROM, and progressive therapeutic exercises to the (L) elbow, wrist, and hand. Will include general ROM and strengthening exercises to the shoulder to minimize effects of decreased activity on that musculature/joint.

Stephanie Wright, PT

Chapter Five

Documentation Practice

Becky McKnight, PT, MS
Mia L. Erickson, PT, EdD, ATC, CHT

CHAPTER OBJECTIVES

After reading this chapter, the student will be able to:

1. List components of the patient/client management model that should be documented in the medical record.

2. Identify tasks that must be documented by the PT and those that can be documented by the PTA.

3. Describe the purpose of the APTA's *Guidelines for Physical Therapy Documentation.*

4. Report basic principles for documentation.

5. Report principles for documenting patient care.

6. Identify components of patient care when given a physical therapy note.

7. Correctly document late entries and appropriately correct errors in medical records.

8. Demonstrate the appropriate guidelines when writing physical therapy notes.

DOCUMENTATION IN PHYSICAL THERAPY

Documentation of physical therapy services occurs over a continuum, throughout a patient's episode of care. Documentation begins with the initial examination, evaluation, and plan of care as performed and written by the PT.

Subsequent documentation includes progress notes or updates for every encounter with the patient. Progress notes can be written by either the PT or the PTA. Progress notes are interim notes written to record treatment sessions and progress toward the goals stated in the initial evaluation. In many cases, the patient's record will also include reevaluations performed and written by the PT. Reevaluations should occur as the patient's status changes, warranting a reevaluation, or within a required time frame as dictated by state law. Final documentation is performed at the summation of care. This is the last entry in a patient's record and is usually referred to as the discharge summary. This note often reflects results of a discharge evaluation, which is also performed and written by the PT.

The entire physical therapy record should reflect: (1) the patient's condition, or pathology; (2) impairments and functional deficits identified through appropriate tests and measurements; (3) anticipated goals and expected outcomes; (4) interventions provided, including patient education, communication with other disciplines, and specific procedural interventions; and (5) the final outcome or result of the intervention. It is the position of the APTA that the physical therapy examination, evaluation, diagnosis, and prognosis be documented, dated, and authenticated by the PT performing the service. Interventions provided by the PT or PTA should be documented, dated, and authenticated by the PT, the PTA (where permissible by law), or both.[7] This record should be kept in a secured file to meet confidentiality requirements.

The APTA has set forth standardized *Guidelines for Physical Therapy Documentation.*[7] The purpose of these guidelines is to "provide (documentation) guidance for the physical therapy profession across all practice settings."[7] While they are not intended to reflect documentation requirements in all specialty areas, the guidelines can serve as a "foundation" for developing documentation procedures across a variety of unique and specialized settings.[7] Other authors have also reported specific guidelines for documenting in medical records.[8,10,18-20,23,27,33,42] This chapter divides documentation principles into 2 parts, Basic Principles and Documenting Patient Care. Basic Principles provides general rules for documenting in medical records, while the second section, Documenting Patient Care, provides more specific details related to how a physical therapist assistant will document an interim note in the SOAP note format.

BASIC PRINCIPLES

- Be *timely*. It is important that documentation is completed as soon after the session as possible. First, the treatment session is fresh in your head, and you are more likely to remember details sooner after the session rather than later. In addition, your documentation might be necessary so that another therapist can treat your patient in the event of your absence. There are also managerial reasons for timely documentation. These include filing reimbursement claims and sending progress updates to others involved in the patient's care including physicians, case managers, or insurance companies. Clinics are likely to have policies in place requiring completion of all patient documentation within a given time frame.

- All entries made in the medical record must be *relevant, thorough, accurate, and logical*. You should be able to examine your records and have an accurate detailed depiction of the patient and situation. Any clinician should be able to pick up one of your patient records and treat the patient in the case of your absence.

- Entries must be *clear and concise*. While it is important to be as concise as possible, you should also be thorough. Never leave out pertinent information for the sake of brevity.

- Be *consistent*. Use similar types of documentation throughout the patient's episode of care at your facility, eg, forms, SOAP format, flow sheets. This allows reviewers and other health care providers ease in locating necessary information.

- Use *objective* language including facts and observations. Avoid making subjective remarks about patients, including anything that can not be substantiated by the data. This includes subjective remarks about a patient's response to a treatment (eg, "tolerated treatment well"), the patient's personality, or his or her psychological status. Also, avoid subjective terms such as "appears" and "seems to be."[28] While you may be trying to provide additional information about the patient, you must be very careful not to make an unsubstantiated judgment.[23]

- Write *legibly*. Third-party payers have been known to deny claims based solely on the fact that they could not read the provider's handwriting.

- Use *black or blue permanent ink*. Ball point is preferred over felt-tip pens. Erasable ink should never be used.

- Use *scientific, medical terminology*. Avoid "non-skilled language" such as "The patient walked..." Use descriptive, functional language instead such as "Provided gait and transfer training...."

- Use only *industry-standard and facility-approved medical terminology, symbols, and abbreviations* (Appendix A). Please note that you should not overuse abbreviations. This can become confusing for the reader, especially if they are unfamiliar with any of the abbreviations. In addition, some abbreviations have more than one meaning (ie, PT = physical therapist and prothrombin time). In these cases, you must read the entire note to determine the context of the abbreviation, so that you can interpret it appropriately. Check with your facility regarding acceptable abbreviations and their use.

- Use of first-person is generally not acceptable. *Third-person* is preferred because the emphasis should be on what the patient can do or does.

  Example:

  Instead of: I ambulated the pt. 50' and provided min (A).

  Use: Pt. ambulated 50' c̄ min (A) x 1.

  However, there are times when it is unavoidable. These are usually when there has been a special situation, and you are describing what happened in the narrative format.

- *Avoid skipping lines* in the record. When writing in a medical record, you should begin your note with the date of service on the line immediately below the prior entry. Do not skip lines between entries. Furthermore, you should not skip lines in the middle of your notes. Skipping lines could allow someone to come back at a later date and fraudulently add information.

- Add *headings*. Make it easy for the reader by grouping relevant information together and using titles and headings. Examples of appropriate headings will be provided later in this chapter. Also, heading use in initial evaluative notes can be seen in boxes 4-6 through 4-8 in Chapter 4.

- In instances where there is a great deal of data that can easily become confusing to the reader, it is appropriate to use *tables, columns, or lists.* Tables are valuable when documenting range of motion or strength on several joints such as the hand. Examples of use of tables or columns will be provided later in this chapter.

- Documenting *late entries:* After completing the documentation for a particular treatment session and placing it in the medical record, a therapist might realize a need to document additional information about the session. The original note should never be rewritten. Instead, the therapist should complete a late entry. The entry should be placed in chronological order for the *date that it is written* and be identified as a "late entry." An explanation for the late entry should also be provided.[33]

- *Correcting errors* in medical records: Indicate an error with a single straight black line through the text. An individual reading the note should still be able to read what was written originally. Initial and date next to the error. Never use correction fluid or erasable ink in a medical record.

  > **Example:** The patient ~~ambulated~~ MLE 2/18/04
  > transferred with min (A) x 1.

- *Date and authenticate* all patient records. All physical therapy records should be dated according to the day the services were provided. Authentication is "the process used to verify that an entry into the medical record is complete, accurate, and final. Indications of authentication can include original written signatures and computer "signatures" on secured electronic record systems only."[7,p703] Signatures should also include the clinician's full name and designation (PT or PTA).[18]

- Document reasons for *cancelled or missed appointments or treatment sessions* whether initiated by the pt. or the PT, the PTA, or another health care provider, eg, in an outpatient clinic, a snow storm in January caused your patients to miss their appointments for 2 days; on a skilled-nursing unit, the nurse asked for therapy to be held in the morning while waiting for a consultation by a psychologist.

- Document all *telephone or internet conversations* related to patient care. This could include conversations with the patent, the patient's family, the physician, other health care providers, or case managers. Currently the APTA is investigating the creation of guidelines for any internet consultation. Eg, you are working with a 24-year-old who was injured in a workplace accident, and the patient's case manager for worker's compensation contacts you to determine the patient's status and progress.

- Document any *unusual or unexpected situations/results.* Some of these situations may also need an incident report completed. Completion of incident reports will be discussed further in Chapter 6 within discussion of legal aspects of documentation. Eg, you are working with a 22-year-old female who underwent an ACL repair. She is performing resisted knee flexion with a pulley system and felt a "pop" in her knee with a moderate increase in pain.

- When documentation of patient care requires *more than 1 page of entry* make sure each page includes the patient's name, the patient's number, and the date. You should transition the information by writing a statement like: PT note for (patient's name and date) continued.

DOCUMENTING PATIENT CARE

When documenting interventions or services provided in an interim note you should include specific descriptions of the intervention and equipment provided. This information is frequently documented through the use of checklists, flowcharts, or graphs. To demonstrate the patient's status (progression or regression) you should document the following types of information:

1. Subjective information that helps to demonstrate the patient's status.

2. Changes in objective and measurable findings as they relate to the initial evaluation and the existing goals.

3. The patient's reaction to treatment (positive or negative).

4. Progression/regression of the treatment plan, including patient education.

5. Communication or collaboration with other health care providers, the patient, and the patient's family or caregiver(s).[1]

Each interim note needs to both refer to the initial evaluation and also be able to stand alone. The information documented in an interim note helps to demonstrate progression of therapy services, as well as the patient's response to those services, so the note needs to be structured to demonstrate how the information refers to the initial plan of care. On the other hand, each note needs to be written as clearly as possible and with enough detail that it can independently support the intervention provided that day (Table 5-1).

Table 5-1

COMPARING WHAT INFORMATION IS FOUND IN AN INITIAL EVALUATIVE NOTE COMPARED TO AN INTERIM NOTE IN THE SOAP FORMAT

	Initial Evaluation	Interim Note

Pr	· Patient's chief complaint
	· Medical diagnosis
	· Physical therapy diagnosis
	· Loss of function
	· Any information gleaned from the medical record
	  ° Recent or past surgeries
	  ° Past conditions or diseases
	  ° Present conditions or diseases
	  ° Results of medical tests
		· Patient's chief complaint
		· Medical diagnosis
		· Physical therapy diagnosis
		· Loss of function
		· New test results

S	· Patient's current and past medical history · Patient's symptoms or complaints · Factors that cause the symptoms or complaints · Patient's prior level of function · Patient's lifestyle/occupation/societal roles · Patient's goals	· Patient's status · Patient's reaction to intervention · New problems or new complaints · Pertinent information not previously documented

O	· Information gathered through:
	  ° Tests
	  ° Measures
	  ° Observation
	· Interventions provided
	  ° Communication/Collaboration
	  ° Patient related instruction
	  ° Procedural interventions
	· Data that demonstrates the patient's response to interventions provided
		· Patient status
		  ° Data collected
		  ° Patient's functional status
		  ° Observations
		· Interventions provided
		  ° Communication/Collaboration
		  ° Patient related instruction
		  ° Procedural interventions
		· Data that demonstrates the patient's response to interventions provided

A	· Physical therapist's interpretation of the S and O data · Identification of impairments and functional limitations · Goals · Physical therapy diagnosis · Prognosis/rehabilitation potential · Justification for goals/treatment plan · Explanation of any difficulties with obtaining S or O data · Suggestions for further testing, treatment or referrals · Summary of the patient's response to interventions	· A summarization of the S & O · Summary of the patient's response to interventions · Reference how the patient is progressing toward the goals established in the plan of care

P	· Plan for intervention activities to occur
	  ° Collaboration/communication
	  ° Pt. related education
	  ° Procedural interventions
	· Frequency/duration of therapy services
	· Treatment progression
	· Plans for further assessment or reassessment
	· Equipment needs
	· Referral to other services
		· What actions need to occur within areas of intervention
		  ° Communication/Collaboration
		  ° Patient related instruction
		  ° Procedural interventions
		· When the next session is scheduled
		· Any equipment or information that needs to be ordered or prepared before the next session

Box 5-1

Example Problem Section of an Interim Note

Anytown Community Hospital
Skilled Nursing Facility

Physical Therapy Progress Note

Patient: D.T.
Date: 04/04/04
Pr: Left Patellectomy; (L) LE ROM & strength deficits

Informed Consent

Informed consent is a method of informing the patient of the treatment or care that you will be providing. Initially, the PT obtains informed consent when discussing the plan of care with the patient. However, you might be required to obtain informed consent when implementing a new modality. In this case, you are required to explain the procedure, determine presence of contraindications, and describe risks and benefits where appropriate.

Problem (P)

The problem section of the SOAP note answers the question, "What is the main problem?" In an interim note you should document the diagnosis or main physical therapy problem. This information helps to provide a context for the rest of the documentation. You can find this information in the initial evaluation. Also in this section you may include results of any new tests or procedures from the medical record such as radiology or lab results (Box 5-1).

Subjective (S)

The subjective section of the SOAP note answers the question, "What does the patient (or the patient's family member/caregiver) have to say?" The subjective information provides the patient's perspective and documents valuable information to support the effectiveness of the treatment plan or demonstrate the need for alteration of the treatment plan. When writing the "S" section you will document any comments from the patient or the patient's family member(s), caregiver(s), or significant other(s) that demonstrates the patient's status/progress, the patient's reaction to interventions provided, new problems or complaints, or any pertinent information not previously documented.

Patient's Status

- Pain rating and description. Eg, a 48-year-old male, who is recovering from a back injury, was asked to rate his pain using a numerical scale of 0 to 10 (0 being no pain and 10 being worst possible pain). The patient currently rates his pain as 3/10 and describes the pain as a "pulling" pain.

- Patient's perception of symptoms. Eg, a 76-year-old male in a skilled nursing facility who is recovering from an exacerbation of COPD, reports, "I am feeling stronger."

- Patient's functional abilities. Eg, a 35-year-old female recovering from complications resulting from a radical mastectomy reports, "I was able to put the dishes into the cabinet last night for the first time since my surgery."

- Statements that demonstrate the patient's cognitive or emotional status. Eg, an 84-year-old female, recovering from an ORIF of a fractured femur, has been a widow for several years and was living alone prior to the accident. While in therapy, the patient comments that her husband is waiting in her room to take her dancing.

- Comments related to accomplishment of goals/outcomes. Eg, you are working with a 32-year-old female who is recovering from a humeral fracture. One of her personal goals is to be able to care for her 10-month-old infant. Today, in the clinic, she proudly reports, "I was able to change the baby's diaper last night all by myself".

Patient's Reaction to Interventions Provided

- Behavior of the patient's pain since the previous intervention. Eg, a 52-year-old female is receiving therapy due to a diagnosis of adhesive capsulitis. The patient states that her pain level increased after her last therapy session when a new stretching activity was initiated, but she reports the increase in pain only lasted about an hour, and then the pain returned to its normal level.

- Comments that demonstrate if the intervention provided is effective. Eg, a 64-year-old male suffering from chronic cervical pain has received a trial of TENS. The patient reports no relief of pain symptoms with the TENS trial.

New Problem(s) or New Complaint(s)

- New pain complaints. Eg, a 77-year-old male patient is recovering from an elective THA. The patient had medical complications and was on bed-rest longer than anticipated, and his recovery has been delayed. As you begin working with him, he comments that his heels have been very sore from lying on the bed so much.

Pertinent Information Not Previously Documented

- Medical history. Eg, you are working in an outpatient setting. You have been assisting with the care of a 48-year-old male who injured his back while moving. Today, as you are working with him, he informs you that he had a hernia repair 2 years ago. You know that this information was not included in the initial evaluation or any of the subsequent interim notes.

- Environment: lifestyle, home situation, work, school. Eg, you have been assisting with the care of a 72-year-old man in a skilled nursing facility. He had a femur fracture and will be NWB for 6 to 8 weeks per the physician's report. The patient's goal is to return home, where he lives alone. You know from the evaluative note that the patient has 4 steps without any railing to enter his home. As you are working with the patient he reveals that his "steps" are nothing more than cinder blocks stacked on top of each other.

Structure/Organization

The subjective data is often highly organized in the initial evaluative note. The physical therapist will often categorize information under subheadings to provide structure to the note and to allow for a logical flow of the information. Subheadings for the information can vary and may be delineated by facility policy. When writing an interim note, it is infrequent that you will need to utilize subheadings. You will want to organize the subjective information by grouping similar information. You will want to keep all information related to the patient's pain (rating, description, and behavior) together, while keeping all information related to the home environment (distance needed to walk, steps to negotiate, type of flooring) together. There may be a few occasions when you will need to document many pieces of subjective information. In this case, you can use subheadings to organize the information. Example subheadings that might be used in the subjective section include:

- Current Condition
- Patient Complaint
- Living Environment
- Functional Status/Activity Level
- Medical/Surgical History
- Family Health History
- Social History
- Employment Status

Box 5-2

Example Subjective Section of an Interim Note

S: Pt. c/o continued weakness in (L) knee. He reports being ambulatory with no assistive device when at home, uses one crutch when on uneven surfaces, outside of the home. He states he has made moderate improvements with therapy.

Tips

When writing the subjective information:

- Indicate exactly who is providing the information, eg, the patient, the patient's spouse, the patient's son or daughter, the caregiver.

- Use verbs like: states, reports, complains of, denies, describes, etc.

- Use quotes to demonstrate the patient's cognitive or emotional status or attitude toward therapy.

- While the first word of the subjective is usually "Pt.", it is not necessary to repeat "Pt." at the beginning of every sentence. Once it is written the first time, it is implied in subsequent sentences.[43](Box 5-2)

Objective (O)

The objective section of a SOAP note answers the questions, "What is going on with the physical therapy intervention?" and "How is the patient responding to the intervention?" Information in this section should be reproducible. In other words, another PT or PTA should be able to provide the same interventions or utilize the same techniques (test/measure/observations) to collect data related to the patient's progress. Objective information in an interim note falls into 1 of 2 categories: (1) Physical therapy intervention provided or (2) Information that demonstrates the patient's response to the physical therapy intervention provided.

Intervention Provided

- Communication and coordination, eg, discussion with nursing staff about the patient's pain medication schedule.

- Patient related instruction, eg, education related to hip precautions with a patient who is recovering from a THA.

- Procedural interventions, eg, transfer and gait training, therapeutic exercise program, physical agents.

Patient's Response to Physical Therapy Intervention Provided

Responses are demonstrated by:

- Data collected. The results of all data collection techniques such as goniometry or manual muscle testing.

- Description of the patient's function. Eg, description of the patient's ability to move around in bed.

- Observations about the patient. Any general observations that can not be categorized as data from a specific technique or a description of function. This may include information such as description of an open wound, description of patient's movement strategies, or documentation of tenderness to palpation.

Structure/Organization of O

There are a number of ways to structure information in the objective section of a SOAP note. The goal is to organize the note to allow the reader to be able to easily find the information and to provide a logical flow. Subheadings are used to organize the information. The choice of subheadings can either be determined by the facility, or it can be left up to the discretion of the physical therapist. If the facility has not established standard subheadings, you should refer to the initial evaluative note to determine which subheadings you will use when you write your interim note. When you have information that does not easily fall within the subheadings noted in the initial evaluative note, you may choose alternative subheadings. Appropriate headings for the objective portion of the note are:

1. Aerobic Capacity
2. Anthropometric Characteristics (ie, girth)
3. Arousal, Attention, and Cognition
4. Balance
5. Circulation (ie, vitals—heart rate and blood pressure, pulses, capillary refill)
6. Cranial and Peripheral Nerve Integrity
7. Environmental, Home, and Work Barriers
8. Ergonomics and Body Mechanics
9. Gait
10. Integumentary Integrity
11. Joint Integrity or Mobility
12. Locomotion (moving from one place to another, ie, transfers)
13. Motor Function
14. Muscle Performance (ie, strength, power, and endurance)
15. Neuromotor Development and Sensory Integration

16. Orthotic, Protective, and Supportive Devices
17. Pain (although verbally stated pain and global ratings are indicated in the subjective portion of the note, eg, Pain Numerical Rating Scales and Pain Verbal Rating Scales)
18. Posture
19. Prosthetic Devices
20. Range of Motion (AROM, PROM, and flexibility)
21. Reflexes
22. Self-Care and Home Management Skills
23. Sensation
24. Ventilation/Respiration
25. Work, Community, or Leisure Status and Integration or Reintegration (including IADLs)*

* For a thorough description of each of these including definitions and tools used for gathering data, see the *Guide for Physical Therapist Practice, 2nd edition.*[7]

Often information in the objective section is best communicated in list, column, or table format. These formats are used to make the information easier to follow. Columns or tables are also used to document comparative data, like previous status beside current status or pre-intervention measurements compared to post-intervention measurements. Information that is frequently documented in this format includes goniometric and MMT results.

Example:	AROM	PROM	*Strength*
(R) Hip Abduction	20°	30°	3-/5
Adduction	0°	10°	2-/5
Flexion	80°	95°	3-/5
Extension	0°	5°	2+/5
(R) Knee	10-100°	5-120°	3-/5
(R) Ankle DF	5°	20°	3-/5
PF	45°	45°	4/5
Inv	20°	30°	3+/5
Ev	5°	15°	3+/5

General Tips

- Document results of tests and measures in the same manner as they were performed and documented in the PT initial evaluative note. Use the same scale used in the initial evaluation.

- Not all information addressed in the initial evaluation needs to be addressed in each interim note.
  - ○ Only address data obtained while reassessing the patient during the treatment session.
  - ○ It is not necessary to address areas that were found to be within normal parameters in the initial examination/evaluation if those areas are still normal.

- Document related to what the patient did, not what the PTA did.
- A copy of any written instructions provided to the patient should be included in the medical record and referred to in the "O" section of the note.
- Complete sentences are not necessary, but information should be clear enough to get the idea across.
- Use verbs like demonstrated, performed, appears, is, etc.

Tips for Documenting Interventions Provided

When documenting interventions provided, include all information that is necessary to reproduce the activity:

1. What intervention was provided, eg, modality, exercise, or gait training
2. Amount of the intervention, eg, dosage, number of repetitions, or distance
3. What equipment was used, eg, TENS, 5 pound weight, standard walker
4. Setting on equipment
5. Specific treatment area
6. Patient positioning
7. Duration, frequency, and rest breaks
8. Anything that would not be considered standard practice

Communication/Coordination
- Supervising physical therapist
- Other health care practitioner, eg, physician, RN, OT, prosthetist
- Administrators/case managers
- Phone conversations with any of the above

Patient Related Instruction
- Therapeutic activity instruction, eg, HEP
- Precautions/restricted activity, eg, total hip precautions or lifting restrictions
- Education related to disease process, eg, What is a stroke?
- Education related to physical therapy procedures, eg, What is US and why is it used?

Procedural Interventions
Functional Training
- Types:
  ○ Activities of daily living
  ○ Assistive/adaptive devices
  ○ Body mechanics
  ○ Developmental activities
  ○ Gait and locomotion training
  ○ Prosthetics and orthotics
  ○ Wheelchair management skills
- Include in documentation:
  ○ Specific activity, eg, bed to w/c transfers
  ○ Assistive/adaptive devices used

Infection Control Procedures
- Isolation or sterile techniques used, eg, use of gown and gloves when assisting with therapy exercise

Manual Therapy Techniques
- PROM
  ○ Extremities/joints
  ○ Number of repetitions
- Massage
  ○ Location
  ○ Type of massage
  ○ Amount of time

Physical Agents and Mechanical Agents
- Types:
  ○ Athermal agents
  ○ Biofeedback
  ○ Compression therapies
  ○ Cryotherapy
  ○ Electrotherapeutic agents
  ○ Hydrotherapy
  ○ Superficial and deep thermal agents
  ○ Traction
- Include in documentation:
  ○ Physical or mechanical agent used, eg, IFC
  ○ Patient position
  ○ Specific area treated
  ○ Exact settings used
  ○ Duration of treatment

Therapeutic Exercise
- Types:
  ○ Aerobic conditioning
  ○ Balance and coordination training
  ○ Conditioning and reconditioning activities
  ○ Posture awareness training
  ○ Range of motion exercises
  ○ Stretching exercises
  ○ Strengthening exercises
- Include in documentation:
  ○ Specific activities/exercises performed
  ○ Equipment used
  ○ Patient position (if not clear by use of equipment)
  ○ Reps/duration

Box 5-3

**Example Objective Section
of an Interim Note**

O: *ROM:* (L) LE   AROM   PROM
Flex   0° to 135°   0° to 140°
Strength:(L) LE   quads 3+/5, hamstrings
4-/5, mild discomfort noticed with knee
extension
Gait: Able to ambulate 250' without assistive device or immobilizer independently but
does display decreased cadence and guard-
ing. Demonstrates abnormal heel (R) toe gait
pattern and has a tendency to keep LE
extended when walking.
*Treatment:*Continue with strengthening exercises for hams & quads. Including proprioceptive exercises to improve stabilization of
the knee.

Wound Management
- Application and removal of dressings or agents
  ◦ Type and amount of dressing used
- Precautions for dressing removal

Equipment Provided
- Eg, theraband for HEP

Response to All Procedural Interventions
- Can be documented in either "O" or "A" (Box 5-3)

Tips for Documenting Results of Data Collected

When documenting results of data collection, include all information needed for the test to be reproduced and for the results to be clearly understood. Be sure to include:

1. Procedure utilized, eg, goniometry, MMT, observation
2. Exactly what was measured, eg, (R) elbow flexion PROM
3. The patient's position

Types of Data Collected

*Vital Signs (indicate before and/or after exercise/
activity as appropriate)*
- Heart Rate
  ◦ Location
  ◦ Quality
  ◦ Rate
- Respiratory Rate
  ◦ Rate
  ◦ Rhythm

◦ Depth
◦ Regularity of pattern
- Blood Pressure
  ◦ Location, side
  ◦ Systolic over diastolic
  ◦ Eg, BP: (R) brachial 120/80

Anthropometrical Characteristics
- Height
- Weight
- Length
- Girth

Muscle Strength
- Range, eg, when documenting strength for (R) elbow flexors document 3/5 instead of 3
- What is measured
  ◦ Muscle group, eg, hip flexors
  ◦ Specific muscles, eg, gluteus maximus
- Arrange logically
  ◦ Group per anatomical location, eg, group shoulder musculature together: shoulder flexors 4/5, extensors 4-/5, abduction 4-/5, adduction 4+/5
  ◦ Use tables or columns to show (B) measurement or before/after measurements
- Any deviation from standard position/protocol, eg, tested hip extension in side lying due to pt. unable to get in prone because of obesity

Pain
- Results from written pain questionnaires, scales, and diagrams
- Examples include: McGill Pain Questionnaire, Pain Disability Index, Visual Analogue Scales, Pain Drawings, and Pain Maps
- Note: verbal descriptions of pain given by the patient are written in the subjective portion of the note

Range of Motion
- Document the range from the beginning of the range available to the end of the range available, eg, elbow flexion 5° to 110° instead of just elbow flexion 110°
- Specific joint
- Arrange logically
  ◦ Group per anatomical location
  ◦ Use tables or columns to show (B) measurement or before/after measurements
- Any deviation from standard position/protocol, eg, shoulder external rotation; unable to achieve standard test position due to pain restrictions; pt. placed in 45° of abduction for measurement

Results of Any Standard Tests or Questionnaires
- Record measurements per the standard of the test being used, eg, Berg Balance Test

Describing Patient Function

Assistive, Adaptive, Orthotic, Protective, Supportive, and Prosthetic Devices
- Specify device being used, eg, (L) custom AFO.
- Discuss pt.'s (pt.'s family/caregiver's) ability to care for device.
- Discuss pt.'s ability to don/doff device as appropriate.
- Discuss skin condition related to use of the device.
- Discuss safety risks associated with use of the device.

Gait, Locomotion, and Balance
- Indicate activity, eg, gait or wheelchair mobility.
- Indicate any assistive, adaptive, orthotic, protective, supportive, or prosthetic devices used, eg, wheeled walker.
- Indicate type of surface the pt. is traversing, eg, level surface or stairs.
- Indicate distance traveled or amount of time activity is tolerated, eg, 100 feet or 10 minutes.
- List amount and type of physical assistance provided, eg, pt. required min (A) to place (L) LE.
- Number of people needed to provide assistance.
- List amount and type of cues given, eg, pt. required constant verbal cues for cane placement.
- Describe gait pattern used if appropriate, eg, 4-point gait pattern.
- Describe gait deviations if appropriate, eg, pt. demonstrated (L) foot drop during swing phase of gait.
- When documenting gait include weight bearing status.

Self-Care, Home Management, and Community or Work Reintegration
- Record measurements of physical environments.
- Record any safety concerns or barriers in home, community, and work environments.

Results of Any Standard Tests or Questionnaires
- Record measurements per the standard of the test being used. Eg, Functional Independence Measure (FIM), SF-36, Disabilities of the Arm, Shoulder, and Hand (DASH).
- *The Interactive Guide to Physical Therapist Practice with Catalog of Tests and Measures* CD-ROM (available from www.apta.org) provides a comprehensive list of assessment tools and references for their associated reliability and validity as reported in the literature.

- Table 5-2 provides an abbreviated list of more common functional assessment tools and their respective patient populations.

Note: In order to provide greater objectivity and reliability when documenting functional status, some clinics and facilities utilize standardized tests or questionnaires to measure impairments, function, and degree of disability. Each test or questionnaire will have specific directions related to appropriate documentation to allow for consistency of administration and scoring. When utilizing a standardized tool, the clinician and facility will want to verify its validity and reliability. Specific tools are designed for specific patient populations. A tool that has been determined to be valid in one setting may not be appropriate in another. Finally, traditional grading of function (independent, minimal assistance, etc) should be consistent with scoring given on standardized instruments. Table 5-3 demonstrates a comparison of documentation of functional status utilizing traditional terminology and scoring utilizing a standardized test for measuring a patient's function, the FIM.

Observations

Arousal, Mentation, and Cognition
- Describe changes in pt.'s state of arousal, mentation, and cognition, eg, pt. lethargic today; difficult to arouse and attend to therapeutic activities.

Integumentary Integrity
- Location of wound/skin condition
- Size of wound
- Depth of wound
- Location and depth of any tunneling/undermining
- Description of tissue
- Description of surrounding area
- Description of drainage
- Description of odor
- Activities, positioning, and postures that aggravate or relieve pain, alter sensation, or produce associated skin trauma

Joint Integrity and Mobility
- Describe abnormal joint movements/end feels.

Muscle Performance
- Describe abnormal muscle mass, eg, (L) LE gastroc atrophy compared to (R) LE.
- Describe change in muscle tone, eg, noted hypertonicity of (R) LE during gait with straight cane.

Neuromotor Development
- Describe gross and fine motor milestones.
- Describe abnormal righting and equilibrium reactions.

Table 5-2

COMMON STANDARDIZED FUNCTIONAL TESTS AND APPROPRIATE PATIENT POPULATION

Standardized Assessment	Patient Population
Acute Care Index of Function (ACIF)	Acute Neurological
Arthritis Impact Measurement Scale (AIMS2)	Arthritis
Asthma Quality of Life Questionnaires	Asthma
Cardiac Health Profile	Cardiovascular Disease
Dallas Pain Questionnaire	Chronic Spinal Pain
Diabetes Impact Measurement Scale (DIMS)	Type 1 and Type 2 Diabetes
Disability Rating Scale	Severe Head Trauma
Fatigue Impact Scale	Chronic Disease
Fibromyalgia Impact Questionnaire	Fibromyalgia
Foot Function Index	Foot Pain
Frail Elderly Functional Assessment	Frail Elderly
Functional Independence Measure (FIM)	Variety
Functional Performance Inventory	Moderate to Severe COPD
Fugl-Meyer Assessment Scale	CVA
Gross Motor Performance Measure (GMPM)	Children with Cerebral Palsy
Gross Motor Function Measure (GMFM)	Pediatric
Harris Hip Scale	Hip Arthritis
Neck Disability Index (NDI)	Neck Disorders
Oswesty Low Back Pain Disability Questionnaire	Low Back Disorders
Parkinson's Disease Quality of Life (PDQL)	Parkinson's Disease
Patient-Rated Wrist Evaluation (PRWE)	Wrist Disorders
Peabody Development Motor Scales	Pediatric Motor Development
Pediatric Evaluation of Disability Index (PEDI)	Pediatric
Physical Disability Index	Frail Elderly
SF-12	Variety
SF-36	Variety
Sickness Impact Profile (SIP)	Variety with Versions for Nursing Home Residents and Stroke
Stroke Impact Scale	CVA
Therapeutic Associates Outcomes System	Variety of Musculoskeletal Disorders
Western Ontario and McMaster Universities Osteoarthritis Index	Osteoarthritis
WeeFIM	Pediatric Function

Pain
- Describe pt.'s non-verbal pain responses to activities, positioning, and postures
- Pain questionnaires

Posture
- Describe alignment of trunk
- Describe alignment of extremities in relation to the trunk

Ventilation, Respiration, and Circulation Examination
- Describe skin color in relation to circulation and ventilation
- Describe symptoms of ventilation/respiratory or circulatory deficiency
- Describe chest wall expansion and excursion

- Describe cough
- Describe sputum color and consistency

Assessment (A)

The assessment section of the interim SOAP note answers the question, "What does it all mean?" This is the PT or PTA's opportunity to explain the relevance of the documented data. A key point to remember about writing the assessment to is to *provide a picture of why skilled services are needed.* This is the PT or PTA's (where allowed by law) opportunity to summarize the patient's progress (or lack thereof), status toward goals, changes in condition, ongoing impairments, functional limitations, and disabilities. This is the place to make obvious how interventions have led to changes in the patient's status.

Table 5-3

HOW DOCUMENTATION OF FUNCTIONAL STATUS UTILIZING TRADITIONAL TERMINOLOGY COMPARES TO FIM SCORES

Term	Abbreviation	Amount/Type of Assistance Needed	FIM Score	Descriptor	Amount/Type of Assistance Needed
Independent	(I)	No assistance needed	7	Complete independence	All of the tasks described as making up the activity are typically performed safely, without modification, assistive devices, or aids, and within a reasonable amount of time
No direct correlation with FIM score	No direct correlation with FIM score	No direct correlation with FIM score	6	Modified independence	One or more of the following may be true: · The activity requires an assistive device · The activity takes more than reasonable time · There are safety risks
Stand-by assist	SBA	Needs someone close by for safety or to provide verbal or visual cues	5	Supervision or setup	Subject requires no more help than stand-by, cuing, or coaxing, without physical contact, or helper sets up needed items or applies orthoses or assistive/adaptive devices
Contact guard assist	CGA	Needs someone touching the patient for safety or to provide physical cues	No direct correlation with FIM scores	No direct correlation with FIM scores	No direct correlation with FIM scores
Minimal	Min	Pt. performs 75% or > of the effort	4	Minimal contact assistance	Subject requires no more help than touching, and expends 75% or more of the effort
Moderate	Mod	Pt. performs 25-75% of the effort	3	Moderate assistance	Subject requires more help than touching, or expends half or more of the effort (50% - 75%)
Maximal	Max	Pt. performs 25% or < of the activity	2	Maximal assistance	Subject expends less than 50% of the effort, but at least 25%
Dependent	Dep	Pt. unable to assist in any way	1	Total assistance	Subject expends less than 25% of the effort

Imagine that you are talking with an insurance company, and you really want to portray the patient's status.

This section will provide a summary of the "S" and "O" information. In these sections you should include an explanation of how the data demonstrates the patient's response to the intervention(s) provided and a statement about how the patient is progressing in reference to the goals established in the plan of care.

Explanation of How the Data Demonstrates the Patient's Response to Intervention

- Change in pain level. Eg, you are providing TENS application for pain control for a patient with chronic back pain with radicular symptoms. Prior to initiating intervention, the pt. rates his pain as 7/10. After initiation of TENS trial the pt. rates his pain as 2/10.

- Change in impairment. Eg, you are assisting with the care of a patient who has lymphedema. You are using volumetric measurements to document amount of edema before and after intervention.

- Change in functional status. Eg, you are working in an outpatient clinic with a 32-year-old male who injured his back playing football with friends. When he enters the clinic, his c/o pain and stiffness caused him to be unable to bend over to take off his shoes. After receiving physical agents and appropriate therapeutic exercise, the patient is able to put on his shoes to leave the clinic.

Patient's Progress Toward Goals

- Whether a goal has been achieved
- Progress toward a goal
- No progress toward a goal
- Decline in patient status

Tips

- There should never be any information in the "A" section that does not relate to data documented in "S" & "O" sections.

- Back up all statements with data from the "S" & "O" sections. Eg, if you document that the patient has an improvement in their mobility, refer to the data documented in the "O" section that substantiates that comment.

- Be specific. Do not document, "Tolerated treatment well" or "Patient progressing." Always indicate how you know these things.

- In keeping with the disablement theme, you should indicate relationships between impairments, function, and disability in this section. For example, the following statement would be very appropriate: A: Patient continues to have decreased AROM in the (R) shoulder limiting her ability to dress and reach into her overhead cabinets.

Box 5-4

Example Assessment Section of an Interim Note

A: Showing improvement in ROM and strength and functional gait. Pt. has met STG's 2 & 3. Will cont. to work toward STG's 1 & 4 and all LTG's.

- The effect of the interventions on impairments, function, and recovery should be highlighted. Eg, A: Pt. demonstrating improved ROM in the (R) shoulder since starting HEP. Improvement in ROM has allowed better ability to dress and reach into overhead cabinets (Box 5-4).

Plan (P)

The Plan section of an interim SOAP note answers the question, "Where do we go from here?" The plan should be based upon the established plan of care and the patient's response to the interventions and progression toward goals. The plan will delineate what actions need to occur within the 3 areas of intervention: (1) coordination/communication and documentation, (2) patient/client-related instructions, and (3) procedural interventions. Types of information that can be included in the "P" section of an interim note include:

- Coordination/Communication and Documentation
  - Request for a reexamination/reevaluation by the physical therapist, eg, the patient is not progressing as desired with the current plan of care/treatment plan.
  - Communication with other health care providers, eg, discussing discharge plans with a social worker.

- Patient/Client-Related Instructions
  - Written instruction to be provided, eg, will issue and instruct in HEP next session.
  - Education regarding activity level/precautions, eg, will educate patient regarding hip precautions and car transfers.

- Procedural Interventions
  - Progression of treatment plan within established plan of care, eg, will increase resistance with therapeutic exercises.
  - Modification of treatment plan within established plan of care, eg, will change from using a standard walker to using a wheeled walker due to the patient's continued problems with appropriate sequencing while using the standard walker.

- ° Equipment to be purchased, eg, wheeled walker for home use.
- ° Activities to perform, eg, will focus on bed mobility training.
- Schedule for continued therapy, eg, to continue with BID treatments with anticipated discharge in 3 days to home.

Tips

- Use phrases such as "Will check...", "Will update...", "Will consult...", "Will increase...", "Will hold..."
- The plan should include anything that you are thinking about doing with the patient.
- This should serve as a reminder to you during the patient's next session and provide a guide for the next therapist or assistant treating the patient (Box 5-5).

Box 5-5

Example Plan Section of an Interim Note

P: Cont. PT in the outpatient setting 3x/wk for strengthening, ROM and proprioceptive exercises, and gait training.

Jody Laughlin, PTA

Now that you know basic documentation principles and specific guidelines for documenting patient care in a SOAP note format, you should be able to adapt and document this information in an appropriate manner regardless of the policies and styles you are presented with in the clinical situations you encounter.

Review Questions

1. Who is responsible for writing the initial examination? Progress notes? Reevaluations? Discharge evaluations?

2. What is the purpose of the *Guidelines for Physical Therapy Documentation*?

3. How much time should elapse between treating a patient and documenting the session?

4. What color(s) of ink are most appropriate for medical record documentation?

5. What does the term "authenticate" mean?

6. Examine the laws in your state (and surrounding states) concerning medical record documentation requirements. What are they? How might they affect you as a PTA?

7. Examine the Physical Therapy Practice Act in your state (and surrounding states). What are the documentation requirements? Are these different depending on the type of facility (eg, hospital, outpatient clinic)?

8. In your state, what components of the physical therapy documentation are PTAs allowed/not allowed to write? Are PT co-signatures required?

APPLICATION EXERCISES

I.   For the following entries, indicate examples that are *inappropriate* by writing an "I" next to the item. Describe why they are inappropriate.

   1. _____   The patient walked 50'
   2. _____   Skilled services are needed
   3. _____   Pt. stated that she enjoys coming to PT
   4. _____   Pt. c/o pain in the (L) knee following exercise p̄ last visit
   5. _____   *AROM:* (R) shoulder flexion 160° abduction 120°
   6. _____   Pt. performed QS, GS, and SLRs
   7. _____   Pt. walked around the PT gym 2x
   8. _____   ROM knee 0-135°
   9. _____   Pt. demonstrating global aphasia
   10. _____ Pt. is demonstrating excessive hip abduction c̄ his prosthesis during ambulation
   11. _____ *Gait:* 100' c̄ hemi-walker c̄ min (A) x 1 for trunk support and min (A) x 1 for advancing the (L) LE
   12. _____ *Transfers:* Bed ↔ chair c̄ min (A) x 1 2° to poor balance
   13. _____ *Ther Ex:* Performed 20 repetitions all exercises
   14. _____ *Bed Mobility:* Rolls supine ↔ SL with min (A) x 1
   15. _____ *HEP:* Instructed the pt. in a HEP to be performed tid

II.   Write the following information in a more clear and concise manner, as it would appear in the medical record.

   1. The patient walked 75 feet in the hallway of the hospital with the therapist lightly touching her back. She used a front-wheeled walker.

   2. The patient's strength was 3/5 for the right biceps and 4/5 for the right triceps.

   3. Upon arrival to therapy, the patient told you that she had been doing her HEP without any problems and really felt like her ability to get in and out of bed had improved.

   4. The patient said that her pain was 3/10 on a pain scale.

   5. You performed ultrasound to the dorsal aspect of the patient's right foot. You used 3 MHz at 50% duty cycle with the intensity set at $1.0 w/cm^2$.

6. The patient demonstrated the following range of motion measurements: active range of motion for the right elbow was 130° flexion and 10° of hyperextension.

7. Knee active range of motion was 100° flexion and lacking 10° of extension.

8. The patient propelled his wheelchair around the hospital, outside on the sidewalk, and up and down several ramps with you providing verbal reminders on trunk positioning for going up and down the ramps.

9. The patient was able to put her ankle-foot orthosis on and remove it independently. She was also able to check her skin for any irritated areas after she removed it.

10. You instructed the patient to perform 10 repetitions of each exercise as part of her home exercise program. The exercises included ankle pumps, quadriceps setting, short arc quadriceps strengthening from 45° to 0°, and heel slides.

11. During a busy morning in a hospital, you were working with a patient who told you that she was going to be discharged and wanted home health services, primarily PT. After writing the note and moving on to the next patient, you realize that you did not document the patient's desire for home PT. What should you do? In the space below, demonstrate how you would document this entry into the chart? Where should this information be placed?

12. When writing the following information in the chart, you realize that you made an error in documenting the patient's AROM. It should have been 125°, not 152°. Demonstrate how to correct this mistake.
    AROM: (R) shoulder flexion 152°

III. Organize the following information so that it is clear, concise, and suitable for entry into the medical record.

1. Mr. Jones comes into the clinic today and tells you that his fingers became swollen and that he has had pain at a level of 7 out of 10 since the last treatment session. He goes on to say that he has not been able to perform any of the range of motion exercises you gave him because of the incredible amount of pain he has been having. He said that he has changed his post-operative dressing once a day, and he has had a little bit of red drainage on the bandages. He also said that he is having trouble eating and shaving due to the swelling and stiffness in the joints.

2. You enter Mrs. Smith's hospital room and ask her if she is ready for treatment. She agrees and tells you that she wants to be ready to walk down the aisle at her grandson's wedding without using her walker. She said that her right knee pain is not as bad as it was yesterday, and she thinks that she is able to bend it more. She goes on to say that she has performed the range of motion exercises twice already this morning, and she is working on trying to get her knee to bend as much as she can. While walking, she asks if she can begin using a cane soon.

3. Mr. Smith comes into the Physical Therapy Department and tells you that he notices improvement in his walking since beginning the active range of motion exercises for his ankle. He also says that he is having 0 out of 10 pain with the new exercises. He goes on to tell you that he still has pain when walking on gravel, carpet, and stairs. His job (logger) requires him to do a lot of walking on uneven terrain, and he wants to be able to do this without pain before returning to work.

4. You are assigned an inpatient who had a right cerebral vascular accident 3 weeks ago. The supervising PT told you that she is demonstrating confusion and slurred speech, but her daughter is usually present during the sessions. Upon entering the patient's room, you notice the daughter is not present. As you work with the patient, she tells you that she fell in the bathroom last night. She also tells you that she is afraid to get out of bed because of her fear of falling again. It was difficult for you to understand the patient due to the slurring. You also understand the patient to say that her left shoulder is sore. While performing bedside active assistive range of motion, her daughter returns, and you comment to the daughter about the patient's fall the previous night. The daughter tells you that there wasn't a fall and that she had been there with her mother all night.

5. While treating a patient during a home health visit, the patient's son tells you that his mother (the patient) has been up all night due to left hip pain. He also tells you that he is having trouble getting his mother to walk in the house with him due to pain and fear of making her hip hurt more than it already does. He also says that he has trouble performing the range of motion exercises that you showed him during the last session. The patient tells you that, because of the pain, she feels like her hip is going to give out when she stands on it.

6. Right knee flexion 100°, right knee extension 5°, hip abduction 20°, hip flexion 100°, ankle PF 20°, elbow AROM 10-100°, shoulder flexion 100°, shoulder abduction 100°, hip IR 20°, ankle DF 5°, shoulder ER 60°, and IR 45°.

7. Walked 10', twice, with one person supplying 25% assistance, used a standard walker, did not put any weight on the right leg, needed verbal reminders each time for placing the walker forward.

8. Up and down 4 stairs with a hand rail that was on the right side going up and on the left coming down; the pt. used a straight cane.

9. The patient walked with the therapist at his side (but not touching him) for 100 feet, twice; vitals signs before exercise were blood pressure 125/85, 15 for respirations, and 77 for heart rate; vitals after were 135/85 for blood pressure, 17 for respirations, and 87 for heart rate; the patient performed ankle pumping, elbow flexion, shoulder flexion, and knee extension for 10 repetitions before and after exercise.

10. Girth at the right knee joint line was 34 cm, 2 inches above was 38 cm, 4 inches above was 42 cm, and 4 inches below was 35.5 cm. Active flexion was 120°. The patient lacked 20° of active extension. Hip and ankle active range of motion were within normal limits. Strength for the quad muscle was 3-/5 and for the hamstring was 3-/5. The patient walks independently with crutches, weight bearing as much as he can tolerate on the involved extremity.

11. You are working with a patient with a diagnosis of bicipital tendonitis in an outpatient clinic. She tells you that she has been working on the home exercises, and overall, her arm is feeling much better. She reports pain to be 3/10 on a verbal pain scale. She says that she has trouble reaching into overhead cabinets and shelves. Her treatment consisted of ultrasound over the anterior shoulder for 6 minutes, 50% duty cycle, with the intensity set at 1.5 w/cm^2. This was followed by gentle active range of motion exercises with a wand for flexion and external rotation, active scapular retraction and protraction, prone horizontal abduction, and external rotation with yellow theraband for 2 sets of 10 repetitions. She also received manual stretching for flexion, internal rotation, and external rotation (performed by you). The treatment concluded with ice for 15 minutes. She reported better ROM and less pain when the treatment was over. She will return 2 times each week for the above treatment and progression of the exercises as tolerated.

12. You are working with a patient 3 days status post right total knee replacement in the PT gym. She has noticeable swelling and limited range of motion in the knee and ankle. She transfers to and from the mat with you providing 25% assistance. She transferred sit to and from supine with you performing 50% assistance due to her inability to lift the right leg onto the mat table. She performed 2 sets of 10 repetitions of the total knee exercises and ambulated 50 feet, twice, with a standard walker, only putting 50% of her body weight on the involved extremity. She received ice for 15 minutes to her knee. You notice that she walked only 25' during yesterday's session. She will be seen in the afternoon for the same treatment, progressing gait as tolerated.

IV. Organize the following information so that it is clear, concise, and suitable for entry into the medical record. Use the initial evaluative note (Box 5-6) that follows when writing the note.

   You have treated the patient today (December 6, 2004) and note the following. Write a progress note based upon this information.

When you enter the room the patient is finishing with his bathing. The nurse helps him to dress in his jogging pants and sweatshirt. You ask if he is ready for therapy. He grumbles a bit but agrees. The patient seems irritated. Upon inquiry he reports that he wants to go home but "you guys won't let me." You respond appropriately to that statement. You assist the patient to the therapy department. Given the choice whether to walk first or exercise first the patient chooses to walk. The patient is sitting on the edge of the bed and has no trouble standing up to his walker. You help the patient walk. He tires after about 75' but he is able to walk with only verbal cues for using his walker appropriately. After the patient takes a brief rest break in a chair, you help him practice ambulating on stairs. The patient has difficulty with the task and needs 25% assistance for walker placement and a boost to raise himself up the steps. He states his shoulders are hurting and that going up the stairs really bothers them. You assist the patient to the therapy mat where he needs assistance to raise his operated limb up onto the mat while laying down. The patient performs all the exercises the therapist previously ordered—2 sets of 10 repetitions each. The patient still required assistance with SLR. The therapist also had asked you to add some shoulder exercises. So the patient performed all shoulder movements with a 2-pound weight for 1 set of 10 repetitions. After the mat exercises, you have the patient sit up. He needs a little bit of physical assistance to get his leg off the mat and to help push his upper body. You then help him to perform standing hip extension and flexion and abduction of his affected limb while holding on to his walker. You assist the patient back to his chair and assist him back to his room telling him you will be back for another session in the afternoon (Box 5-6).

Box 5-6

Anytown Community Hospital
Skilled Nursing Facility

Physical Therapy Evaluation

Patient: I.H.
Age: 67 y/o
Date: 12/03/04
Referral: Physical therapy for gait and strengthening. Anterior hip precautions, WBAT.
Referring Physician: Dr. Mark John

Pr: Pain and DJD (L) Hip s/p THA

Hx: This 67 y/o patient was admitted for a THA 11/30/04. PMH includes DJD bilateral shoulders, HTN, and two previous TIA's approx. 1 year ago.

S: *Complaint:* The patient states he does have general soreness but his hip pain is less than before the surgery. Rates pain as 1-2/10.

Living Environment/Social Support: The patient lives at home with spouse. Has 3 steps with railing to enter his one level home. The patient states his hobbies include yardwork and doing crossword puzzles.

Prior Level of Function/Activities: The patient was previously (I) with shoulder level and below ADL's and gait without (A) device.

Goals: The patient wants to return to his normal level of functioning.

O: *ROM:*

Hip	(L)	(R)
Flexion	0° to 30°	0° to 135°
Abduction	0° to 0°	0° to 30°
Shoulder		
Flexion	0° to 90°	0° to 95°
Abduction	0° to 75°	0° to 80°

Peripheral Vascular Assessment:

Color	slight pallor; refill brisk	pink
Temp	toes slightly cool	warm
Touch	intact	intact
Pulses-Dorsalis Pedis	regular; slight diminished	regular and full

Girth: (L) 3cm> (R) 8cm at the center of the patella

Strength: 4/5 to 4+/5 throughout (B) UE's and (R) LE except shoulders 3+/5. (L) hip MMT deferred 2° to recent surgery; appears 2/5 with functional mobility. (L) knee strength 3+/5, ankle strength 5/5.

Mobility: Scooting in bed with min (A), Supine ↔ Sit with Mod (A), Sit ↔ Stand with min (A).

Gait: Pt. ambulated 50' with walker and min (A) WBAT (L) LE. Pt. needed frequent v/c's for proper walker placement. Pt. had a tendency to place walker too far in front of him. C/o mild discomfort in shoulders with using walker.

Intervention: Initiated AAROM to (L) LE. Pt performed ankle pumps, quad sets, ham sets, glut sets, SAQ, SLR, hip abd, and heel slides 1 x 10.

Pt. Education: Pt. was instructed in hip precautions and was given a written reminder sheet of precautions.

continued

Patient: I.H.

A: Pt. is very motivated and has excellent rehab potential. Extremity segment, peripheral vascular check, and ROM all within post-THA limits.

Problem List:
1. Decreased strength (L) LE
2. Dependent mobility
3. Dependent gait
4. Hip precautions

STGs: To be met within 2 days
1. Increase (L) LE strength to 3-/5 throughout hip and 3+/5 knee
2. Pt. will require SBA-CGA with all bed mobility & transfers
3. Pt. will ambulate 100' c̄ walker & CGA on level surfaces
4. Pt. will be able to verbalize hip precautions

LTG's: To be met within 7 days
1. Increase (L) LE strength to 3+/5 throughout hip and 4/5 knee
2. Pt. will be (I) c̄ all bed mobility & transfers
3. Pt. will ambulate 200' c̄ walker (I) on level surface & up and down 3 steps with SBA
4. Pt. will display good understanding of hip precautions during all functional activities

P: PT BID for transfer and gait training, ROM/strengthening exercises, and education regarding hip precautions.

Mary Good, PT

Chapter Six

Reimbursement Basics

Mia L. Erickson, PT, EdD, ATC, CHT

CHAPTER OBJECTIVES

After reading this chapter, the student will be able to:

1. Define reimbursement.
2. Differentiate between first, second, and third-party payers.
3. Differentiate between different types of insurance (social, managed care, casualty, and indemnity).
4. Explain the difference between Medicare Part A, Medicare Part B, and Medicaid.
5. Examine Medicare reimbursement in a variety of settings (inpatient hospitals, inpatient rehabilitation hospitals, skilled nursing facilities, home health care, and outpatient facilities).
6. Examine strategies for cost containment utilized by managed care organizations.
7. Construct a physical therapy progress note using basic principles for maximum reimbursement.
8. Realize how documentation is tied to reimbursement.

WHAT IS REIMBURSEMENT?

There are generally 3 parties involved in the financial management of an individual's medical care: (1) the patient (first party); (2) the health care provider, such as the physician, physical therapist, occupational therapist, etc (second party); and (3) the insurance company (third party). When a patient receives a service from a health care provider, some form of payment is expected. This payment can come directly from the patient (first-party payment), but more often it comes from the patient's insurance company. Payment to the health care provider from the insurance company is known as third-party payment, or reimbursement. The APTA has defined reimbursement as the payment received by a health care provider from an insurance company or other payer (ie, government agency, employer, state worker's compensation fund) for performing a service for a patient.[44] Third-party payment accounts for more than 80% of all payments for rehabilitative care.[45] The financial success and viability of physical therapy departments and clinics is usually dependent upon reimbursement from insurance companies or third-party payers. In the past, providers were paid, or reimbursed, 100% of what they billed the insurance company. Today, however, this is not the case. Now there are many rules and regulations governing the amount of money paid to providers for their services, and they vary according to different insurance companies, payers, and insurance policies.

TYPES OF INSURANCE

As you begin your clinical affiliations and begin to practice as a PTA, you will realize that there are many types of insurance. There are many differences in the benefits provided by these insurers as well. A brief description of common types of insurance is provided in this chapter. For more detail, the APTA's *Reimbursement Resource Guide* provides an extensive overview of different types of insurance and reimbursement guidelines.[45]

Social Insurance

Social insurance is a type of insurance where money is directed from individuals who can pay to those who can not. Examples are Medicare, Medicaid, and state programs for individuals who do not have health insurance.[45]

The Social Security Act of 1965 established Medicare and Medicaid to provide the elderly and the poor with health insurance coverage. In 1972, Medicare benefits were extended to individuals with disabilities and those with permanent kidney failure.[46] Today, Medicare provides benefits to[21]:

1. People 65 years of age and older who are receiving or eligible for Social Security Retirement benefits.

2. Younger individuals with disabilities who meet the Social Security Act's requirements for disability.

3. Individuals with end-stage renal disease (ESRD) (ie, permanent kidney failure with dialysis or transplant).

From 1977 to 2001, Medicare and Medicaid services were coordinated under the Health Care Financing Administration (HCFA). In 2001, HCFA changed its name to the Centers for Medicare and Medicaid Services (CMS).[47] Today, CMS administers and manages traditional Medicare, Medicare beneficiary options, and state programs such as Medicaid and SCHIP (State Children's Health Insurance Program). CMS is a federal agency housed in the Department of Health and Human Services.

Medicare

Medicare is a federally funded program that consists of 2 parts—Medicare Part A and Medicare Part B. Medicare Part A, or Hospital Insurance Part A, pays for inpatient hospital stays, skilled nursing facilities (SNF), hospice, and some home health care. It does not cover long-term care or nursing homes. Medicare beneficiaries (individuals who receive Medicare benefits) do not pay a fee for Medicare Part A. This payment came from monthly payroll deductions while the individual was employed. Also, enrollment in Part A is automatic for individuals receiving Social Security benefits.[48] Medicare Part B, or Medical Insurance Part B, pays for physician services, outpatient services, durable medical equipment (DME), and some services not covered under Part A, like physical and occupational therapy. Enrollment in Medicare Part B is optional. In order to receive benefits under Part B, individuals are required to enroll and pay a monthly premium ($66.60 in 2004 and $78.20 in 2005). This amount is deducted from their monthly Social Security benefit payment.[48]

For Parts A and B, home health care, and DME, Medicare contracts with private insurance companies to pay the bills. For Part A and some Part B, these companies are known as fiscal intermediaries (FI), or intermediaries.

For Part B, they are known as carriers.[21] Regional home health intermediaries (RHHIs) pay bills for home health care and monitor its quality, and durable medical equipment regional carriers (DMERCs) pay bills for durable medical equipment. These fiscal intermediaries and carriers are determined based on geographic regions. It is important to know the payers for your region so that you can become familiar with their reimbursement and documentation guidelines, as they may differ. The following Web site: http://www.cms.hhs.gov/contacts/incardir.asp#4 provides a listing of fiscal intermediaries and carriers for each state as well as a link to its Web site.

Medicare reimbursement varies depending on the type of facility in which you practice. Different payment systems are in place for different practice settings. Prospective payment systems (PPS) are in place for acute care hospitals, inpatient rehabilitation hospitals, SNFs, and home health care. PPS is a type of Medicare reimbursement based on a predetermined, fixed amount.[21] The payment amount is derived from patient classification systems specific to the setting (acute care, rehabilitation, SNF, etc). Upon admission to one these facilities or services, patients are "grouped" according to common characteristics such diagnosis, disease, and functional status. These are known as case-mix groups. For each case-mix group, Medicare has agreed to reimburse a predetermined fixed amount.[49] The facility's admissions data, or in some settings, data from standardized evaluation tools, are used to assign patients to a case-mix group.

PPS in inpatient acute care hospitals is known as Inpatient PPS, or IPPS. Under the IPPS, each patient is categorized into a diagnosis-related group (DRG). A DRG is a classification system used to group patients according to diagnosis, type of treatment, age, and other relevant criteria.[21] Hospitals are paid a set, predetermined amount according to the patient's DRG category, regardless of the actual cost to provide care to the patient.[21] More information about IPPS and DRGs can be found at http://www.cms.hhs.gov/providers/hipps/default.asp.

Reimbursement provided to SNFs is based on a PPS, but in these facilities, the amount Medicare pays is determined through information provided by each patient upon his or her admission. For each patient entering a SNF, a minimum data set (MDS) assessment is completed. This is a multidisciplinary assessment performed by a variety of health care providers (physician, physical therapist, occupational therapist, speech therapist, nurse, etc) that includes data such as ADL status, nursing needs, behavior, and cognitive status.[50] Data from the MDS is then used to determine the patient's Resource Utilization Group, version III (RUG-III), classification. The RUG-III classification is a hierarchy for grouping patients according to the amount of resources they will need during their stay at a

SNF.[50] For example, more complex patients require more staff resources; therefore, facilities are reimbursed at a higher rate. There are 7 major RUG-III classifications. They are: rehabilitation, extensive services, special care, clinically complex, impaired cognition, behavioral problems, and reduced physical functioning. For more information on each of these categories, you can go to http://www.cms.hhs.gov/medicaid/mds20/rai1202 ch6.pdf.

Reimbursement to inpatient rehabilitation facilities (IRF) is similar to that of a SNF, with a few exceptions. Upon admission to an IRF, patients are assessed using an Inpatient Rehabilitation Facility Patient Assessment Instrument (IRF PAI). These data are used to classify patients based on clinical characteristics and anticipated resource needs.[51] Payments are determined based on the patient's classification. The Functional Independence Measure (FIM) is an integral part of the IRF PAI for rehabilitation practitioners in these settings. The FIM is administered on all patients in this setting, and the scores are used as data on the IRF PAI.

Patient case-mix groups in home health care are also determined by assessing data collected during the admissions process, like SNFs and IRFs. However, in home health, the assessment tool is known as the Outcome and Assessment Information Set (OASIS).[49] Data from the OASIS is used to categorize patients into 1 of 80 Home Health Resource Groups (HHRG), and payment is predetermined for each group. While the OASIS is not meant to serve as a comprehensive assessment tool, it does require information on the patients' "sociodemographic, environmental, support system, health status, and functional status attributes."[52] The OASIS is also used for home health agency quality improvement and tracking patient outcomes.

As you can see, each setting has unique assessment tools, categories, and guidelines for reimbursement by Medicare. It is important to point out that while reimbursement has been predetermined for each of the case-mix groups, payments can be adjusted based on geographic location and cost of providing services to particularly complex patients. Reimbursement can also be adjusted for teaching hospitals and to providers who treat a large number of patients without insurance. This is known as case-mix adjustment.

Reimbursement provided to hospital-based, physical therapy outpatient clinics and physical therapy private practices is based on the Medicare Physician Fee Schedule (MPFS). The MPFS is the PPS for physical, occupational, and speech therapy provided in this setting. Fee schedules are pre-determined lists of payment amounts for various services performed by physicians or health care providers.[21,44] This predetermined amount is also known

as the "Medicare allowable." For example, according to the APTA Web site, the Medicare allowable for a physical therapy evaluation is ~$72.00. It is important to point out that in outpatient settings, Medicare will reimburse 80% of the Medicare allowable. The remaining 20% is the patient's responsibility. The remaining 20% is often paid by the patient's secondary insurance, except in cases where the patient does not have secondary insurance. Then the remaining 20% must be paid by the patient. The APTA provides a link to an up-to-date Medicare fee schedule to its members on its Web site at http://www.apta.org/ Govt_Affairs/regulatory/Medicare.

The Medicare allowable is determined through the use of an elaborate coding system. First, all health care procedures are assigned a code under the Current Procedural Terminology (CPT). This is known as the procedure's CPT Code. Under the CPT system, physical therapy procedures begin with "97." Several examples of physical therapy CPT Codes are:

CPT:	Physical Therapy Procedure:
97001	Physical Therapy Evaluation
97010	Hot pack or Cold pack
97012	Mechanical traction
97022	Whirlpool
97035	Ultrasound

Each of the CPT Codes is then assigned a weight based on: (1) provider work value to administer the procedure, (2) the practice expense, or how much it costs to perform a procedure, and (3) the professional liability (malpractice) value.[45] The professional liability value can be thought of as the associated risk involved with administering a procedure. For example, a joint mobilization has a higher weight than application of a hot pack or cold pack, because a joint mobilization requires more technical skill and has higher associated risk. The scale used for weighting the procedures is known as the Resource-Based Relative Value Scale (RBRVS). Each CPT Code corresponds with an RBRVS Value.

Once the RBRVS value has been determined, it is multiplied by a conversion factor ($37.3374 in 2004).

Hypothetical Example:
Physical Therapy Evaluation (CPT Code 97001)
RBR Value x Conversion Factor = Medicare Allowable
1.99 x $37.3374 = $74.30

After the conversion factor is applied, the dollar value is then adjusted for the geographic region, and that becomes the Medicare allowable for the procedure.[45] In addition to Medicare, other third-party payers use the CPT coding system and the RBRVS to establish fee schedules. Nevertheless, the amount reimbursed by Medicare might vary (higher or lower) with the amount reimbursed by private, non-government insurance companies.

Medicaid

Medicaid is a joint federally and state-funded program that pays for medical care for individuals and families with low incomes and resources. It is the largest source of funding for medical and health-related services for people with limited income.[53] In order to receive Medicaid benefits, certain eligibility requirements must be met. Some of these requirements include being 65 and older, pregnant, blind, disabled, have a low income, and being a United States citizen or lawfully admitted immigrant. Children 18 and younger might also be eligible for Medicaid benefits if certain criteria are met. In addition to these federal regulations for Medicaid eligibility, each state might have its own specific requirements. For a complete overview of Medicaid eligibility requirements, you can access the following Web site: http://www.cms.hhs.gov/medicaid/whoiseligible.asp. Reimbursement provided by Medicaid is different from Medicare and varies from state to state. You should become aware of Medicaid reimbursement guidelines in your state.

For both Medicare and Medicaid, there are some procedures that may be denied coverage. If a health care provider believes that a patient would benefit from a procedure that may not be covered *and* the patient agrees to pay for it, the provider must have the patient sign an advance beneficiary notice (ABN). The ABN must be signed on the day the service is provided. An ABN serves to provide and verify communication to Medicare and Medicaid beneficiaries of their financial responsibility for services that could be denied. In situations where a provider is certain that a procedure will not be covered, the provider must require the patient to sign a Notice of Exclusion of Medicare Benefits (NEMB). Downloadable copies of an ABN and a NEMB are available on Medicare's Web site.[54]

Managed Care

Managed care is a type of health care in which the insurance company (payer) maintains some control over costs and utilization by various means.[44] In the past, physical therapy providers could submit a bill and expect to be reimbursed 100% of the amount billed. However, that is not the case today. With the rise of managed care, health care providers have noticed a reduction in the amount or percentage they are reimbursed. In addition, managed care has created more barriers for health care providers who are seeking reimbursement for their services. The following list provides examples of strategies managed care organizations use to control money paid to providers in order to contain costs.

1. Limiting the number of providers a patient can use—At one time, a patient could choose any provider for his or her health care needs. Now, managed care plans enroll providers into a "network." Patients must then choose from providers within this network. Patients who choose to go outside the network of providers must pay additional costs not covered by the insurance company. These are also known as point-of-service plans. Additionally, in point-of-service plans, patients may be required to "seek primary care from their primary care provider (PCP)."[45] In these plans, the PCP is the point of access into the health care system. The PCP can then direct the patient's care or refer the patient to a specialist. When patients are referred to a specialist through their PCP, they are provided maximum insurance coverage. However, if they enter the health care system through a non-PCP, their amount of coverage is reduced. PCPs can be general medicine, family medicine, or internal medicine practitioners. They can also be pediatricians or, in some cases, gynecologists/obstetricians.[45]

2. Limiting the amount of payment to providers—As indicated previously, in the past, a health care provider could expect to be reimbursed a large percentage of the amount billed. Now insurance companies set limits on how much they will pay providers by implementing a fee-for-service plan, or a fee schedule, similar to the one described for Medicare.

3. Requiring prior authorization—The provider must contact the insurance company (payer) *prior to providing a service* and outline the treatment/services he wishes to carry out. The insurance company may or may not give the provider authorization to perform the recommended service. When prior authorization is required, the insurance company does not reimburse services performed that have not been previously approved. Payment for DME used by PTs and PTAs often requires prior authorization.

4. Limiting the number and duration of services provided—Some insurance companies have policies where there is an established limit on the number of physical therapy visits that will be reimbursed. In addition, there might be language stating that services must be provided within a given time frame.[55] Depending on the insurance, there is a large range and a variety of stipulations. For example, a patient might be allowed 6 visits per diagnosis or 25 visits per calendar year, regardless of diagnosis. There are also cases where the patient is allowed 60 visits in a lifetime. Finally, other plans might allow an initial visit(s) and then require prior authorization from the insurer when additional visits are necessary.[55] You should become familiar with guidelines of frequently encountered insurance companies in your setting.

5. Requiring a utilization review process[21]—Utilization review is an examination of medical necessity, economic appropriateness, and quality of care provided to patients by a health care provider. Reviews may be conducted either by an internal staff person, a committee, or an external independent review organization.

6. Requiring case management[21]—Case managers direct patients to the most appropriate amount, duration, and type of health services and monitor medical outcomes. Insurance companies may employ case managers or contract with an independent case management agency.

Preferred Provider Organizations (PPO) and Health Maintenance Organizations (HMO) are examples of managed care organizations. A PPO is an insurance plan where health care providers contract with an insurance company to treat policyholders according to a predetermined fee schedule. PPOs can range from one hospital and its practicing physicians who contract with a large employer, to a national network of providers that contracts with insurers or employers. PPO contracts typically provide discounts from standard fees, incentives for plan enrollees to use the contracting providers, and other managed care cost-containment methods.[56] With PPOs, patients are covered for care received outside their "network" of providers; however, it is at a reduced rate.[45]

An HMO is a medical group practice plan that acts as both an insurer and a health care provider. Group participants are entitled to services from participating physicians, clinics, and hospitals for a flat monthly or quarterly fee.[56] In an HMO, patients who receive care outside their "network" (except with prior authorization or in the case of an emergency) have no insurance benefits.[45]

Casualty Insurance

Casualty insurance, such as worker's compensation and auto accident insurance, is insurance for individuals who are injured on-the-job or in a motor vehicle accident.[45] These claims are usually handled by payers other than health insurance companies. Worker's compensation plans are run by state governments, and reimbursement and benefits vary from state-to-state. You should become familiar with your state's worker's compensation guidelines for physical therapy reimbursement. The APTA[45] identifies http://www.comp.state.nc.us/ncic/pages/wcadmdir.htm as a useful Web site for investigating worker's compensation laws and agencies in the United States and Canada.

Indemnity Insurance

Indemnity insurance reimburses the patient for their out-of-pocket medical expenses that are covered under the insurance policy. In other words, the patient pays the provider out-of-pocket and submits a claim to his or her insurance company. The insurance company then reimburses the patient. In the case of indemnity insurance, the insurer doesn't provide payment to the health care provider; instead, the contract is between the patient and the insurance company.[45]

DOCUMENTATION AND REIMBURSEMENT

In 1966, Medicare and Medicaid began requiring physicians and other health care providers to document medical procedures in order to be reimbursed.[10] In 1997, Baeten[17] indicated that documentation is the "key to securing reimbursement." This still holds true today.[45]

Physical therapy documentation should include the physical therapist's initial examination, evaluation, and plan of care. Progress notes, reevaluations (as necessary), and a final discharge summary should follow the initial evaluation. The primary documentation role of the PTA is writing progress notes. To maximize reimbursement, progress notes *must*:

1. Reflect a comparison between the patient's current functional status and his or her functional status at the initial evaluation.[57]

2. Include impairments, functional limitations, and degree of disability in clear, concise, objective, and measurable language.[57]

3. Maximize the use of objective tests and measures and avoid terms such as "increased strength."[45,57]

4. Distinguish between verbal and physical assistance.[57]

5. Include regular patient updates,[57] ie, tests and measurements (range of motion, strength) and functional status (gait, transfers, ADLs, and IADLs) should be provided throughout the progress notes, not just on the evaluations and reevaluations.

6. Provide patient updates in a manner consistent with those on the initial evaluation,[57] ie, tests and measurements performed throughout the episode of care should be consistent with those performed during the initial examination (See Chapter 4: The Physical Therapy Process).

7. Indicate why progress might be slower than expected, ie, in the presence of comorbidities.[57]

8. Provide adequate information to support medical necessity of each treatment/procedure on every date it was billed.[57]

9. Provide evidence that unique services of a therapist (skilled services) are required. This includes recording patient's response to treatment and recommending a reevaluation for changes to the treatment plan when necessary.[57]

10. Include the time spent delivering each service.[57]

11. Include a description of the service provided in language that is consistent with what is billed.[45,57]

When documenting, you should always keep in mind that payment could depend upon what you write in the progress notes. It is not enough to write "Pt. improving," "tolerated well," or "skilled services needed." Key points you should always make include: (1) the ongoing need for skilled interventions and (2) how those interventions bring about functional improvement.

REVIEW QUESTIONS

1. In your own words, define reimbursement.

2. Who are the different "parties" responsible for the financial management of a patient's medical care? What is meant by third-party payment?

3. Describe the 4 types of insurance outlined here (social, managed care, indemnity, and casualty).

4. What are the major differences between Medicare Part A and Medicare Part B?

5.   What is the difference between Medicare and Medicaid?

6.   What strategies are used by managed care organizations to contain or lower costs? Give a brief description of each.

7.   Talk with a local clinician about different types of insurance often accepted by their facility. What are their reimbursement guidelines? Try to get examples of managed care plans, Medicare, and Medicaid.

8.   Complete the following table.

Facility	Type of PPS	Patient Categorization	Assessment
A. Acute Care Hospital	_____	_____	_____
B. _____	_____	_____	OASIS
C. _____	_____	RUG-III	_____
D. Inpatient Rehab Facility	_____	_____	_____

APPLICATION EXERCISES

I. Which of the following progress notes best meets the criteria for reimbursement? Why?

S: Patient reporting improvement in her ability to wash her hair and dress with the left arm. Reports pain as 3/10 with excessive overhead activities and at night.

O: *AROM:* left shoulder flexion 130°, abduction 120°. Treatment consisted of 30 minutes of therapeutic exercises to increase shoulder range of motion, including 20 reps of wand exercises for flexion, external rotation, internal rotation, and abduction, manual stretching in the above directions, pulley for 5 minutes, and finger ladder for 5 minutes.

A: Exercises allowing improved ROM. AROM improved 45° since initial visit. Increased motion allowing improved self-care. Patient achieves greater manual stretch from therapist than through self-stretch.

P: Continue with above program with progression per plan of care as stated on initial eval.

Sally Smith, PTA

S: Continues to report night pain and when reaching overhead.

O: Increased AROM; Performed 30 minutes of active and passive exercises to improve joint range of motion.

A: Tolerated well.

P: Continue above 2x/week.

Sally Smith, PTA

S: Patient complains of pain with excessive overhead activities and at night. Having trouble sleeping.

O: *AROM:* left shoulder flexion 130°, abduction 120°. Treatment consisted 20 reps of wand exercises for flexion, external rotation, internal rotation, and abduction, manual stretching in the above directions, pulley for 5 minutes, and finger ladder for 5 minutes.

A: AROM improved since initial visit.

P: Continue with above program.

Sally Smith, PTA

Chapter Seven

Legal and Ethical Considerations for Physical Therapy Documentation

Mia L. Erickson, PT, EdD, ATC, CHT

CHAPTER OBJECTIVES

After reading this chapter, the student will be able to:

1. Describe federal legislation related to privacy and confidentiality.
2. Discuss clinic requirements under the HIPAA Privacy Rule.
3. Compare ethical and legal responsibilities for maintaining confidentiality.
4. Define fraud and abuse.
5. Explain the purpose of risk management.
6. Realize the importance of informed consent.
7. Give reasons for filing an incident report.
8. Outline different agencies' responsibilities in establishing rules for documentation.

INTRODUCTION

As previously indicated, documentation will be one of the most important aspects of your job. When individuals consider becoming a PT or a PTA, they generally do not realize the documentation requirements or their importance. After being in practice for several years and treating a variety of patients, it will become impossible to recall details of each encounter with a patient. Therefore, the information you record while details are fresh in your head will be your reference material if ever necessary. You should document so that if you read the chart several years later, you can recall the patient.

While a full review of legal and ethical requirements and implications for medical record keeping is beyond the scope of this chapter, it should provide an overview of important legal and ethical matters relevant to physical therapy documentation that influence day-to-day PTA practice. These are patient privacy and confidentiality, fraud and abuse, and medical malpractice.

PATIENT PRIVACY AND CONFIDENTIALITY

The Privacy Act of 1974 (5 U.S.C. § 552a)

The Privacy Act of 1974 (http://www.usdoj.gov/foia/privstat.htm) set forth federal guidelines precluding health care agencies or providers from releasing or disclosing medical records or medical information to any person without first obtaining written consent, or a written request, from the patient. The Privacy Act required providers and their employees be trained on rules for handling an individual's records, and administrative efforts were aimed at minimizing threats to maintaining patient confidentiality. This legislation also allowed the patient the right to obtain a copy of his or her medical records (charges can be applied) and discuss the records with his or her provider in the presence of another individual of the patient's choosing. Failure to comply with this Privacy Act would result in civil action against the provider.

In a clinical environment, it is important to maintain and respect the privacy and confidentiality of all information related to patients and clients. When working, you should take care not to leave charts in open areas, accessible to people walking by, and you should be careful not to dictate in an open area where you can be heard by others. Charts should also be kept in a secure locked location so they are not accessible to unauthorized individuals. Clinics and hospitals are also likely to have policies preventing you from taking medical records out of the building. While the Privacy Act of 1974 still holds true today, additional legislation has been passed to further restrict release of an individual's health information and medical records, including those transmitted via electronic media.

Health Insurance Portability and Accountability Act

The Health Insurance Portability and Accountability Act (HIPAA) of 1996 (PL 104-191) required the Department of Health and Human Services (DHHS) to implement standards for performing electronic health care transactions. While electronic transmission of information, including billing and claims filing, was meant to simplify some of these processes, it also increased risks of violating patient privacy and breaching confidentiality. In response, Congress mandated HIPAA provisions to protect personally identifiable health information.[58]

Effective April 14, 2001, the DHHS provided its final regulation, known as The Privacy Rule. The ruling allowed agencies that conduct electronic health care transactions 2 years to come under compliance with standards to protect against the misuse of identifiable health information. Agencies that fail to comply after the effective date, April 14, 2003, are subject to both civil and criminal penalties.[58]

Health care providers, health plans, and health care clearinghouses are subject to the rule if they transmit protected health information through any type of media, including electronic, oral, written, or facsimile. Protected health information includes both personal health information and individually identifiable health information. Electronic media refers to the Internet, intranets and extranets, leased lines, dial-up lines, private networks, or transmissions occurring through magnetic tape, disk, or compact disk.[36]

In addition to protecting identifiable health information, the Privacy Rule requires providers to: (1) make available to patients both written and posted explanations of privacy rights, (2) allow easier patient access to medical records (although charges may be applied), (3) provide employee privacy training, and (4) appoint a privacy officer. Under the Privacy Rule, however, providers are allowed to supply information to insurance companies and third-party payers when seeking reimbursement, and they are permitted to discuss information with other health care providers who are caring for the patient, without any additional written consent from the patient. Information provided to these entities should be on a "minimum necessary" basis, meaning that providers should only disclose the "minimum necessary" information relevant to accomplish the purpose.[36]

The standards apply to health care providers in both the private and public sectors (ie, private and government-run hospitals).[59] However, worker's compensation programs, disability benefit programs, and providers of school-based services under the Individuals with Disabilities Education Act (IDEA) are exempt from the Privacy Rule. Although, these entities are able to adopt the protections if they choose to do so.[36]

Privacy and State Law

At the present time, 48 states have legislation in place regarding privacy of medial records. The Privacy Rule does not replace any state laws, nor does it preclude states from having more restrictive legislation for protecting patient privacy. HIPAA's Privacy Rule merely provides minimum acceptable standards for maintaining and protecting patient privacy.[59] You should investigate the privacy laws in your state as they may differ.

Privacy Recommendations and Computerized Documentation

Maintaining privacy and confidentiality of electronic medical records can be accomplished in several ways. For example, computer systems maintaining patient records should be password protected and secured to prevent unauthorized use and assure private transmittals.[36,60] The American Medical Association recommends assigning different security levels to differing degrees of data sensitivity to limit who has access to the information.[60] Finally, there must be a process for backing-up and storing records.[36,60]

Privacy and Ethics

It is important to understand the difference between ethical and legal responsibilities. Simply stated, ethical responsibility is generally determined by professional associations through development and implementation of a Code of Ethics. Legal responsibilities are determined by both state and federal laws, and failure to comply with the law can result in civil and/or criminal action. You should also realize that unethical behavior or conduct is not always illegal. On the other hand, illegal conduct is usually unethical. Your ethical responsibilities as a PTA have been identified in the *Standards of Ethical Conduct for the Physical Therapist Assistant* and interpreted in *The Guide for Conduct for the Physical Therapist Assistant*. Standard 2, Part 4 (Confidentiality), indicates that information related to patient-client management can not be communicated or provided to a third party without the individual's prior written consent, subject to applicable law. *The Guide for Conduct for the Physical Therapist Assistant* also states that requests for medical records should be directed to the PT.[61] Therefore, in addition to federal legislation and state law, you have a professional ethical responsibility to maintain patient privacy and keep confidential all information related to patients and the care you provide.

FRAUD AND ABUSE

Each year, Medicare and its beneficiaries pay millions of dollars toward fraudulent claims.[62] Insurance fraud can be defined as billing an insurance company, Medicare, or other third-party payer for services that were never provided or billing for an item or service that has higher reimbursement than the service provided.[21] Fraud is a crime and is punishable by law. The U.S. Department of Health and Human Services, the Inspector General, The Federal Bureau of Investigation, and the Department of Justice take part in preventing and detecting Medicare fraud.[62] Accurate billing with corresponding documentation can help prevent fraudulent accusations.

Insurance fraud is both illegal and unethical. Standard 7 of the *Standards of Ethical Conduct for the Physical Therapist Assistant* and *The Guide for Conduct for the Physical Therapist Assistant* put forth the PTA's responsibility in "(protecting) patients and the profession from unethical, incompetent, and illegal acts."[41,61] Keeping with this responsibility, it is also the PTA's duty to report any unethical or illegal acts, including knowledge of fraudulent billing practices.[61]

Another improper billing procedure is abuse. Abuse is when a provider bills for items that are not covered or misuses billing codes.[21] Abuse differs from fraud in that abuse is usually a result of an error or unawareness of the proper code(s) or coding procedure(s). The terms fraud and abuse are often used interchangeably; however, they are very different. To avoid "abusing" the system, you should stay informed of reimbursement guidelines for insurance companies or payers that you encounter frequently.

RISK MANAGEMENT

A growing concern in litigious times and societies is risk management. In this context, risk is defined as the possibility of becoming subject to a liability claim with resulting financial or professional loss(es).[63] Facilities are likely to have risk managers, or risk management departments or committees, whose responsibilities include minimizing potential risks for therapists (PTs and PTAs) who are involved with patient-client management. These individual(s) investigate complaints or concerns as they are brought forth, usually by patients. An important aspect of their investigation is examining the patient record and available documentation. The documentation allows the risk manager(s) to "determine if the care provided met the standard of care required of prudent health care providers."[63]

Price[63] outlined 2 important risk management documents, informed consent documents and incident reports. Informed consent is when a patient agrees to or rejects a specified treatment after being provided with a clear, thorough explanation of its risks, benefits, and treatment alternatives, when available. Additionally, the patient must be provided with information on the probability of success of the treatment as well as the consequences of no treatment at all.[63,64] The PT is ethically responsible for obtaining informed consent prior to providing any intervention. However, the PTA might need to obtain informed consent if initiating a new modality or exercise, as instructed by the PT. Therefore, it is critical to be aware of the patient's previous medical history and current pathology. It is necessary to stay abreast of literature describing indications and contraindications of various interventions you will be providing. You should be able to recognize and communicate contraindications to treatment to the supervising PT. In addition, you should be able to describe to patients the risks, benefits, and alternatives to interventions you perform.

An incident report is a document completed when there is an "incident" that could likely result in a lawsuit. The goal is to document "errors and departures from unexpected procedures or outcomes."[65] A report prepared by the University of California at San Francisco outlined 3 categories of critical incidents needing to be recorded, should they occur. These categories include adverse outcomes to a treatment that has been provided, procedural breakdowns, and catastrophic events.[65] Examples in physical therapy include patients falling during gait training, accidental burns from hot packs or other modality, confidentiality breaches, or any other event that has potential to harm a patient or visitor within or around the hospital or clinic. Incident reports are filed with the risk management department, not in the patient's medical chart.

ESTABLISHING DOCUMENTATION REQUIREMENTS

Federal Agencies

The Centers for Medicare and Medicaid Services (CMS), the government agency that manages Medicare and Medicaid, has set forth a policy requiring health care facilities seeking reimbursement from Medicare and

Medicaid to maintain documentation to support services provided and billed. However, this is CMS's requirement and can only be applied to Medicare and Medicaid. Nevertheless, private insurance companies or other reimbursing agencies can and have adopted similar requirements. In addition, Joint Commission on Accreditation of Health Care Organizations (JCAHO) requires facilities it accredits to maintain medical records for each patient.

State Practice Acts

PTs and PTAs are bound by practice acts in the state(s) where they provide care to patients. Each state has different provisions for PT and PTA practice, some more restrictive than others. The state practice acts often outline provisions for PTA documentation. For example, the Code of Maryland Regulations (COMAR), Title 10, Section 38.03.02-1 (http://www.dsd.state.md.us/comar/10/10.38.03.02%2D1.htm) states that the PTA can document subjective comments, procedural interventions (exercises, modalities, etc) and their parameters, objective functional status, response to treatment, and continuation or changes in the plan as authorized by the PT.

The Federation of State Boards of Physical Therapy (FSBPT) has provided a Web site with links to state licensing agencies and state practice acts. This can be found at http://fsbpt.org/licensing/index.asp. You should become familiar with the practice act for any state where you provide elements of the patient-client management model. In *A Model Practice Act for Physical Therapy*, the FSBPT set forth an exemplary practice act outlining professional conduct and standards for individuals engaged in physical therapy practice.[66] This serves as a model to which state practice acts can be compared. In addition to the FSBPT's Web site, state laws can be found at http://findlaw.com/casecode/#statelaw.

American Physical Therapy Association

The American Physical Therapy Association (APTA) has put forth many recommendations for appropriate documentation. These include their official position statement: *Documentation Authority for Physical Therapy Services*[67] and the *Guidelines for Physical Therapy Documentation*,[7] which has been referred to throughout this text. In addition, *PT—Magazine of Physical Therapy* often provides information on documentation, functional outcomes reporting, computerized documentation, risk management, and liability awareness. The APTA Web site also provides clinicians with useful up-to-date information regarding documentation, including a link to frequently asked documentation questions (http://apta.org/PT_Practice/For_Clinicians/documentation).

While the national association represents physical therapy practitioners across the country, it is important to point out that the documentation guidelines set forth by the APTA are only to serve as a guide. Physical therapy providers (PTs and PTAs) must be first and foremost in compliance with their state practice acts before implementing APTA recommendations. In addition, APTA guidelines are dynamic and tend to change as the scope of practice evolves, while state practice acts change less frequently. It is your professional responsibility to stay attuned to important recommendations from the APTA; however, from a legal perspective, complying first to state laws where you practice is necessary to maintain licensure.

REVIEW QUESTIONS

1. What guidelines did the Privacy Act of 1974 establish?

2. What was the rationale for developing the HIPAA Privacy Rules?

3. What are the requirements for health care providers under the HIPAA Privacy Rules?

4. How do HIPAA's Privacy Rules affect state law?

5. What is your ethical responsibility regarding confidentiality and documentation? Is this different from your legal responsibility? Why or why not?

6. Differentiate between fraud and abuse. Give an example of each.

7. What are your ethical responsibilities related to fraud and abuse?

8. Define risk management.

9. What is the role of risk managers?

10. How is documentation important to risk managers?

11. When seeking informed consent from a patient, what are the key pieces of information that should be provided to the patient?

12. Give 3 examples (other than those listed in the text) of when a PTA would need to file an incident report.

13. What state and federal government organizations are responsible for setting federal guidelines for medical record documentation?

14. To what document(s) can you refer to find laws regarding physical therapy documentation in your state?

15. Investigate the laws for documentation in your state according to your practice act. Do the same for surrounding states. How are they similar? How are they different? How do they compare with the FSBPT's Model Practice Act?

Chapter Eight

SOAP Notes Across the Curriculum

The goal of SOAP Notes Across the Curriculum (SNAC) is to provide you with more examples and practice. SNAC is organized by topics frequently covered in a PTA curriculum. This includes a variety of physical therapy content areas. Each topic or section provides additional documentation problems for you to work through. There are 3 different types of problems. There are problems that will only require you to rewrite a few pieces of information to make them consistent with SOAP note format. There are examples where you will be given an entire treatment session, and you will have to rewrite the information, making an entire SOAP note. Finally, there are examples where you will have to come up with the "A" and/or "P" sections of the note based on the available information or after referring to the initial evaluative note. In all cases, you should write clearly and concisely, using appropriate abbreviations, symbols (Appendix A), and medical terminology. You can use this section all at once during the documentation unit or throughout your program, as you cover the different content areas. Your instructor will guide you on how he or she wants you to complete this section.

Physical Therapy content areas included in SNAC:
- Goniometry
- Strength Assessment
- Range of Motion Exercises
- Transfers
- Tilt Table
- Wheelchairs
- Gait Training
- Wound Care
- Chronic Obstructive Pulmonary Disease/Vital Signs
- Traumatic Brain Injury
- Cerebrovascular Accident
- Lower Extremity Amputation/Prosthetic Devices
- Musculoskeletal Trauma
- Pediatrics/Orthotic Devices

Goniometry

For each of the following, rewrite the information so that it would be appropriate for recording into a SOAP note. Include S, O, A, and P where appropriate.

1. You are working on increasing range of motion in a patient who had a right bimalleolar fracture. After taking the following measurements, you decide that her range of motion goal has been met, and she should be reevaluated by the PT. Active range of motion on the right ankle was 10° of dorsiflexion and 50° of plantarflexion. This is comparable to the left which has 15° dorsiflexion and 55° plantarflexion.

2. You take the following measurements from a patient who is 3 weeks status-post right cerebrovascular accident with left hemiplegia. Active range of motion on the right upper and lower extremities is within normal limits. However, on the left, range of motion is decreased, including: shoulder 45° flexion and abduction, 40° internal rotation, 60° external rotation, elbow flexion 100° and extension 0°, wrist extension 0° and flexion 50°. The left lower extremity demonstrates hip flexion 120°, abduction 20°, knee flexion 130° and extension 0°, ankle dorsiflexion 0° and plantarflexion 50°.

3. The following measurements were taken from a patient on 6/21/04. Active range of motion: right wrist flexion 50°, extension 60°, supination 45°, pronation 45°, ulnar deviation 10°, and radial deviation 5°. On 6/24, you record the following measurements for the same patient. Active range of motion: right wrist flexion 62°, extension 65°, supination 55°, pronation 60°, ulnar deviation 15°, and radial deviation 10°. Organize the measurements for the note on 6/24. Also, what would your assessment be for that day?

4. You are working with a patient who has multiple sclerosis. You record the following measurements. AROM measurements: taken at the ankles: 0° dorsiflexion and 50° plantarflexion, at the knees: extension –20° and flexion 135°, hip flexion was 100°, and hip abduction was 20°. PROM: ankles: 20° dorsiflexion, knees: 0° extension and hips: 120° flexion.

Strength Assessment

Rewrite the following information so that it would be appropriate for recording into a SOAP note. You will need to assign the appropriate muscle grade(s) based on the description provided.

Your supervising PT has asked you to collect data on the following patient's strength. Your findings are below.

1. When assessing a patient's right upper extremity, he is able to take moderate to strong resistance in all muscle groups except abduction and lateral rotation where he is only able to take moderate resistance. Also, he is able to take strong resistance with elbow extension.

2. When assessing the patient's right lower extremity, he is able to take minimal resistance with hip abduction; minimal to moderate resistance with hip flexion, hip extension, and hip lateral rotation; moderate resistance with knee flexion; moderate to strong resistance with hip adduction, knee extension, and ankle dorsiflexion; and strong resistance with ankle plantarflexion.

3. When assessing the patient's left upper extremity, you must use the gravity-eliminated position for all testing. The patient is able to complete full range in this position (he is only able to complete 25% of the range in the gravity-resisted position) and takes some resistance for shoulder adduction and medial rotation. The patient is only able to move through approximately 50% of the available range of motion in the gravity-eliminated position when testing shoulder flexion, shoulder extension, shoulder abduction, elbow extension, and grip testing. The patient is able to complete full available range of motion in the gravity-eliminated position for elbow flexion. You are only able to palpate contractions for the shoulder lateral rotators and the wrist flexors and extensors.

4. When assessing the patient's left lower extremity, he was able to take minimal resistance in the gravity-resisted position when testing hip extensors, hip adductors, and hip internal rotators. He was able to complete full active range of motion and maintain the test position against gravity for hip flexors and ankle plantarflexors. He was unable to complete full range of motion against gravity (only 75%) with hip external rotators and knee extension. He was able to complete only 50% of available range of motion in the gravity-eliminated position for the hip abductors. Only a palpable contraction could be noted with knee flexors and ankle dorsiflexors.

Range of Motion Exercises

Organize the following information into SOAP format.

1. You are working in the acute hospital setting with an elderly female who has suffered a (R) CVA. The supervising therapist has asked you to assist with part of this patient's therapy today. The patient is cooperative and has no complaints. You performed passive and active assisted range of motion to the patient's left extremities. The patient was not showing any signs of abnormal tone or signs of developing contractures. You performed 3 sets of 10 repetitions. You also provided manual resistance to the patient's right lower extremity. The patient tolerated 2 sets of 10 repetitions for the resisted range of motion. Finally, you provided stretching to the patient's tight ankle plantarflexors. You provided the stretch 5 times for each side holding each stretch for 30 seconds. You will continue the same treatment the following day and progress as instructed by the PT.

2. You just finished working with a patient receiving home health care who had a total knee replacement 10 days ago. She was in her bed and performed exercises to work on range of motion. She said she had some pain during the previous night, and she continues to have swelling that she feels is preventing her from bending her knee more. Her biggest complaints right now are not being able to sit normally, go up and down stairs, or drive due to the range of motion limitations in the knee. Her active motion at the knee was 10° of extension and 95° of flexion. You had the patient perform 20 repetitions of heel slides, ankle dorsiflexion and plantar flexion, short arc knee extension exercises, and active hip abduction and adduction. You also worked on active-assistive range of motion to improve knee flexion while the patient was seated at the edge of the bed. She ambulated 50' times 2 with close supervision, weight bearing as tolerated on the right with a standard walker. She stated that she felt good after the exercises. You tell her that you will see her in 2 days to continue the exercises and progress them as she can tolerate.

Answer the following questions about the information below:

- What pieces of information would you examine here to determine the patient's response to the intervention? (See Chapter 5)
- Where would this response be found in the note?

3. You are working with a patient who had a rotator cuff repair 8 weeks ago. During the last session, you initiated resistive range of motion exercises (isometric setting) to begin strengthening the deltoid. He returns to the clinic today and tells you that he has felt good since his last treatment and thinks that the isometric exercises are getting too easy. He thinks that he is able to dress and perform self-care with greater ease. He also notes improved ability to reach into overhead cabinets. After consulting the plan of care, you decide to progress the patient to using an exercise band. While in the clinic that day, he begins shoulder flexion and internal and external rotation using the yellow exercise band. He also performs his usual routine including 20 repetitions of flexion and external rotation with a wand, scapular retraction and protraction, and active external and internal rotation in the side lying position. You also perform 20 repetitions of passive range of motion for flexion, internal and external rotation, and abduction. After the treatment, he said he felt good and thought the new exercises were not that hard. He will return next week, and his exercises will be progressed per the rotator cuff protocol and as he is able to tolerate.

Transfers

For each of the following, rewrite the information so that it would be appropriate for recording into a SOAP note.

1. The patient moved from the bed to the chair with 25% assistance provided by 1 therapist. The stand pivot transfer was used.

2. The patient moved from the wheelchair to the floor using both of his upper extremities with verbal cuing from the therapist.

3. The therapist transferred the patient in the Hoyer lift from the bed to the wheelchair.

4. The patient moved supine to sit and sit to supine with 50% of the assistance provided by the therapist.

5. The patient required 50% of the therapist's assistance when moving from the wheelchair to the mat table when transferring to the left (squat pivot transfer); however, she could transfer to the right with only 25% of assistance provided by the therapist.

6. Your client is a 58-year-old female who has suffered a compound fracture of the (R) ankle. She is NWB on the affected side and is wearing a plaster cast, immobilizing the foot and ankle. The patient is obese and requires moderate assist of 2 people for transferring in and out of bed to a wheelchair. You are to teach her how to transfer effectively from the wheelchair to the bedside commode. She says that she is in severe pain and is hesitant to participate. While using a walker, she was able to stand and doff her pants with minimal assistance but still required moderate assistance of 2 people to complete the transfer to the bedside commode due to fear of falling and difficulty maintaining NWB status.

Organize the following information into SOAP format.

1. You are working with a 68-year-old female who is recovering from a brainstem CVA. Slideboard transfer training with this patient has not gone well. The patient has made poor progress over the last 2 weeks, and the focus of treatment has changed to educating the husband on how to care for his wife. The supervising therapist has asked you to begin Hoyer transfer training with the patient and her husband. The patient is disappointed that she has not made any significant improvements, but she continues to be motivated and "up beat" with therapy. She has stated that she is "not going to give up." The husband required moderate assistance placing the Hoyer sling and setting up for the transfer and needed minimal assistance during the transfer. The patient will be discharged to home with her husband as soon as he is able to care for her independently.

2. You are working with a 28-year-old patient who is in rehab due to a T4 SCI with paraplegia. During this therapy session, you concentrated on working with the patient on his slideboard transfers. The patient was able to perform wheelchair set up with minimal assistance and occasional verbal cues but required moderate assistance with slideboard placement. The patient required maximal assistance with the transfer. The patient shared with you during therapy today that he is concerned about his family and how he was going to manage caring for the farm. The patient appeared depressed and anxious during this session. While looking at the initial evaluative note, you notice there is a goal for the patient to be independent in slideboard transfers.

3. You are working with an inpatient with Guillain Barré syndrome. He reports that he is doing better today. Exercises (3 sets of 10 reps) consisted of ankle pumps, active hip abduction, heel slides, bridging, and knee extension at the edge of the bed. After exercises, you worked on transfers to the wheelchair, which was positioned next to the bed using a stand pivot transfer. The patient required about 25-30% assistance from you, but you were able to provide this yourself without difficulty. Although you did have to block his knees so they did not buckle due to weakness. After this, the patient transferred back to bed, but because of fatigue and bed height, he requires 50-60% assistance. He performed sit to and from supine with 50% assistance because of weakness. He was unable to lift his legs onto the bed from the floor. He was able to position himself in bed without the use of side rails while scooting and bridging with verbal cues. There was no improvement in the patient's ability to transfer from the previous day's note. You tell him you will see him in the afternoon for gait in the therapy department.

Tilt Table

For each of the following, rewrite the information so that it would be appropriate for recording into a SOAP note.

1. You are helping a 78-year-old patient who requires maximum assist from 3 to 4 people to stand. The therapist decides to begin standing activities on the tilt table. The patient has been sitting up in a wheelchair without any complaints or problems. The patient is able to tolerate getting to a full up-right position and stay for 10 minutes before complaining of fatigue. The patient's BP readings remained 120/74 for the full 10 minutes.

2. You are working with a 28-year-old patient who has a closed head injury and exhibits severe hypertonia. The therapist tells you to use the tilt table to help manage lower extremity spasticity. The patient tolerates the procedure without a change in BP (110/76). The patient remains in the upright position for 20 minutes.

3. A 67-year-old who is recovering from a lengthy illness associated with acute respiratory failure, is having consistent problems with orthostatic hypotension. The patient has had 2 previous tilt table treatments and was able to get up to approximately 45° before her BP dropped significantly. At 0° it was 108/68. At 45° it was 92/58 after 1 minute.

Wheelchairs

For each of the following, rewrite the information so that it would be appropriate for recording into a SOAP note.

1.   The patient worked on wheelchair propulsion on ramps and level surfaces for 30 minutes, including tile and carpet, and he is now able to propel independently on all surfaces and manage leg rests and brakes without cuing.

2.   You are working with a 16-year-old patient with a T1 spinal cord lesion. The patient currently needs moderate assistance to perform transfers to and from the w/c with a slideboard. The patient currently requires occasional v/c's and minimal assistance to set up the slideboard and prepare the wheelchair's arm and leg rests for safe mobility in and out.

3.   The patient is 24-year-old and was involved in a MVA and sustained (B) femur fx's. The patient has undergone (B) ORIF and is now being taught slideboard transfers from wheelchair to and from the bed. The patient requires moderate assistance for board set up and minimal assistance for managing the wheelchair parts. She needs moderate assistance from 2 people to transfer in and out of the wheelchair.

4.   You are working with a 58-year-old patient with diabetes, a (R) AKA, and a (L) BKA. The patient has been assigned the following FIM scores. Write the objective portion of your note so that levels of assistance correspond with the FIM scores. Bed, chair, and wheelchair transfers = 3; toilet, tub, and shower transfers = 2; wheelchair mobility = 4.

Organize the following information into SOAP format.

You are working with a patient who has a T3 complete spinal cord lesion with resultant paraplegia. He has been working on the slideboard to transfer in and out of his wheelchair. Currently he is requiring minimal assistant from the therapist (you) to set up and prepare the chair. He requires moderate assistance for the transfer. The ultimate goal is that he will be independent. You spend about 20 minutes on transfer training. He has also been working on wheelchair mobility including ramps, gravel, sidewalks, and carpet. He can perform all of these mobility skills with verbal cuing for weight shifting and occasional minimal assist for trunk control. The goal for wheelchair mobility is also for independence (an additional 10 minutes is spent on wheelchair mobility). For the last part of the treatment session (20 minutes) you work on transferring from the wheelchair to the floor. He requires minimal assist to go to the floor, but requires maximal assist to get back into the chair. This goal is also for him to be independent. You notice on the initial evaluative note that the patient required maximal assist of 2 people for all transfers and moderate assist of 1 person for wheelchair mobility skills when he was admitted to the facility. The plan is to see him twice a day—in the morning for the above and in the afternoon for strengthening, stretching, and continued functional mobility.

Gait Training

For each of the following, rewrite the information so that it would be appropriate for recording into a SOAP note.

Parallel Bars

1. You are to help a 76-year-old obese patient who underwent (B) TKA to ambulate in the parallel bars. She is able to ambulate 10' with moderate assistance of 1 person.

2. An 82-year-old patient with a (R) BKA is beginning gait training with his new prosthesis in the parallel bars. He is able to ambulate 20' with minimal assistance of 1 person.

3. A 45-year-old patient with multiple sclerosis has (B) lower extremity weakness, coordination problems, and balance deficits ambulates 20' in the parallel bars with moderate assistance from 1 person and verbal cuing for upright posture.

Crutches

1. You are to assist a 46-year-old patient who underwent an arthroscopic surgery on his (L) knee ambulate with crutches. He is allowed to weight bear as tolerated and needs minimal assistance for ambulation on level surfaces (for 30 feet) and up and down 2 steps.

2. You are assisting a 26-year-old patient who suffered a (R) femur fracture to ambulate with crutches. The patient is non-weight bearing on the (R) lower extremity. The patient is slightly unsteady but only requires minimal assistance on level surfaces and up and down steps. The patient can ambulate for 50 feet before requiring a rest break.

3. You are working with a 38-year-old patient with multiple sclerosis who recently underwent a (R) TKA. The patient has used loftstrand crutches for years. You are assisting the patient in ambulating with the loftstrand crutches. The patient requires moderate assistance and is allowed to weight bear as tolerated. She can ambulate 25 feet before requiring a break due to fatigue. She has considerably decreased endurance and becomes short of breath easily.

Cane

1. You are assisting a 64-year-old patient with (R) CVA to ambulate with a hemi-cane. The patient requires moderate assistance to ambulate 50 feet. She requires assistance to advance her left leg.

2. You are assisting a 78-year-old patient, who suffered a (L) humerus fracture and is having some mild balance deficits, in learning to ambulate with a straight cane. The patient requires minimal assist due to balance deficits to ambulate 150 feet.

3. A 64-year-old patient who underwent a (R) THA 6 weeks ago is ready to advance from using a walker to using a cane. After instructing the patient, you decide he required contact guard assistance and verbal cuing for proper sequencing.

Walker

1. You are assisting a 74-year-old patient who recently underwent a (R) THA in learning how to ambulate with a walker. The patient requires moderate assistance and is allowed to weight bear as tolerated to walk 75 feet.

2. You are assisting an 84-year-old patient who fell and suffered a (R) wrist and (R) femur fracture. The patient underwent a (R) femur ORIF and is partial weight bearing on the (R). You are to assist her in ambulating with a (R) platform walker. She requires moderate assistance for 25 feet and reminders that she can only place 50% of her weight on the involved lower extremity.

3. You are assisting an 88-year-old patient who is recovering from pneumonia. She is deconditioned and has mild balance problems. Her endurance is poor so she is only able to ambulate 25' before tiring and requiring a rest break. The patient only requires minimal assistance and uses a wheeled walker.

Organize the following information into SOAP format.

1. You are assisting a 28-year-old male who underwent an open reduction internal fixation surgery for a fractured femur. You are assisting this patient with crutch gait on level surfaces and steps. The patient ambulates 300' on level surfaces and up and down 2 flights of steps independently and safely. The patient is ready for discharge. He voices that he wants to go home and is confident he will be able to handle himself. You reference the initial evaluation and note the patient has met all the goals established by the PT. He will be discharged to home in the next 1 to 2 days, and you think that home health would be a good idea for this patient.

2. You are working with a 67-year-old who underwent a left total hip replacement. You see the patient 2 days after the initial evaluation in the skilled nursing facility. Today the patient walked with the walker 100 feet on a level surface and only required contact guard assist. At the time of the initial evaluation, the patient needed minimal assistance. You also began stair training. The patient walked up and down 5 steps with the rail and the walker and required constant verbal cues for sequencing and minimal assistance. The patient voices that he feels he is ready to go home. The goals are for the patient to be independent with gait 200 feet and on stairs since he will be home alone. You will continue to work on advancing him in gait and stairs so that he can return home.

3. You have been working with a 72-year-old male who is recovering from a (L) CVA. The patient has improved his balance to the point that you are now working on gait in the parallel bars. The patient gets easily fatigued and is only able to take 5 to 6 steps at a time. The patient requires maximal assistance to ambulate and needs assistance advancing and placing his right leg. The patient voices that he is sure he will never be able to walk again and says, "we are wasting our time."

Wound Care

For each of the following, rewrite the information so that it would be appropriate for recording into a SOAP note.

1. Upon removing the dressing, you notice minimal to no drainage on the dressing. The drainage there is yellow exudate.

2. The wound bed is necrotic and is entirely filled with black eschar.

3. The area around the wound is red. It also feels warm. It is shiny, and there is also no hair around the wound.

4. After removing the previous day's dressing you notice a "sweet" odor and a moderate amount of greenish drainage on the dressing.

5. Wound is 4 cm in length and 2 cm in width. The depth is 3 mm. There is tunneling 5 cm at 12:00, toward the head.

6. The wound is located at the distal aspect of the lateral leg, just below the lateral malleolus. It has a moderate amount of reddish brown drainage. It is 2 cm by 2 cm with no significant depth.

7. The wound is located on the top of the right foot. Edema is present in the foot and ankle. Figure 8 Girth at the ankle is 20 cm on the right and 16 cm on the left. The periwound area is painful, red, and warm to touch. The dorsal pedal pulse is present and is 1+ on the right and 2+ on the left.

8. The wound is on the anterior aspect of the left tibia. It is 3 cm in length and 4 cm in width. The depth is 5 mm. The wound is full thickness and irregularly shaped. It has 50% granulation and ~25% yellow slough. Part of the tibia and anterior tibialis are exposed. There is no odor present. Sensation is decreased to light touch on the left from the knee down. The treatment consisted of a warm water soak and dressing change using a hydrocolloid dressing to cover the wound.

Organize the following information into SOAP format.

You have been assigned a patient with a diagnosis of Stage 3 open wound at the head of the right first metatarsal, Atherosclerosis, and diabetes mellitus. The patient complains of severe pain and has difficulty walking. There is a minimal amount of non-malodorous reddish brown drainage from the wound bed. The wound bed is moist and has ~50% granulation tissue and 50% yellow adhered slough. The skin around the wound is red, warm to the touch, shiny, and swollen. The wound is a 4 cm x 2.4 cm oval-shaped wound. It is 1.5 cm deep. She has diminished sensation to light touch when compared bilateral. She is unable to feel the 6.65 monofilament on the right. Girth at the right MTP joints is 22 cm and 18 cm on the left. The (R) Dorsal Pedis Pulse is present but diminished compared to the (L) which is 2+. Treatment consisted of WP at 98°F x 15' to (R) LE followed by debridement of a minimal amount of yellow slough from wound bed. After the treatment, the wound was covered with saline soaked gauze and wrapped with kling. It appears to you that the amount of yellow slough in wound bed is decreasing. The initial evaluative note states that there was ~75% yellow adhered slough when the patient began the episode of care. Although there is not much change in wound size. The plan is to continue with the above treatment and try to have the patient begin ambulating as she is able to tolerate.

Chronic Obstructive Pulmonary Disease/Vital Signs

Organize the following information into SOAP format.

You have been assigned a 74-year-old female with a diagnosis of deconditioning and chronic obstructive pulmonary disease. The treatment plan from the evaluative note (performed yesterday) states that the patient will be seen twice daily for endurance exercises and gait training. Upon entering the room, the patient is holding an oxygen mask to her face and taking deep inspirations and short expirations. She complains of difficulty breathing and moving around because she "can't get her breath." She is on 8L of O_2 at rest. Vital signs check before activity reveals the following: pulse 98 bpm, BP 120/84, respirations 20 per minute, O_2 sat 92%. She agrees to participate in bedside exercise, and you spend 15 minutes working on her upper and lower extremities, assuring her O_2 sat levels stay above 90%. After a rest break, she ambulates 30 feet from her bed to and from the bathroom. She requires the O_2 mask with oxygen levels set at 8L during gait. She requires supervision during toileting secondary to complaints of dizziness. She returns to her bed and transfers sit to supine with moderate assist. After exercises and gait, her vitals are: pulse 108 bpm, BP 124/84, respirations 24 per minute, O_2 sat 90%. During the initial examination/evaluation, the patient was unable to ambulate because of her shortness of breath, and her vitals were: pulse 104 bpm, BP 120/88, respirations 24 per minute, O_2 sat 90% at rest.

Based on information provided above, what should be written in the "A" and "P" sections of the note?

Traumatic Brain Injury

Organize the following information into SOAP format.

Your patient is a 72-year-old female with a diagnosis of right subdural hematoma due to a fall. She is alert and cooperative but disoriented to person, time, and place. She is unaware of her situation. Her treatment consisted of bedside exercises including right UE elbow flexion and extension with yellow theraband 2 x 10 and AAROM with the left UE including shoulder flexion and abduction, elbow flexion and extension, wrist flexion and extension, and finger and thumb flexion and extension. You also performed PROM to the (L) hand for increasing the web space ROM. Right LE exercise included hip flexion, extension, ab- and adduction, ankle PF and DF, and knee extension and flexion with yellow theraband 2 x 10. She demonstrated hypertonia on the left upper and lower extremities that increased with speed of movement. There is no abnormal posturing at rest, but she demonstrates a flexion synergy in the left upper extremity with purposeful movements. You also worked on bed mobility including rolling to the right and left and bridging activities. She needs minimal assist x 1 for bed mobility activities. Supine to sit, the patient required minimal assist x 1 also. Stand pivot transfer to the right was performed with minimal assist x 1 and to the left with moderate assist x 1. Sit to stand is with contact guard assist. The patient ambulated 50' x 2 with minimal assist x1 for advancing the left LE and to maintain balance. She has increased extensor tone in the left lower extremity when placing the ball of her foot on the floor. She used a wide base quad cane. She needs reminders for sequencing the steps with placement of the assistive device. She shows poor awareness to safety with gait activities. Overall, you feel that she has been progressing with her program, and she has met several goals for gait distance and transfers. You think that she would benefit from continuing PT at home once discharged and decide to ask the PT for a reevaluation since she has been progressing so well. You are concerned with her lack of safety awareness and question whether the patient's husband will be able to provide adequate care for her once in the home. You decide to mention this to the PT as well and recommend someone being with them for a while in the home once discharged.

After writing the note, answer the following questions:

- What additional information could you include that would improve your note?

- Are there any other recommendations you could make for this patient at this time based on the information provided?

- How has your note met/not met the criteria necessary for reimbursement (Chapter 6)?

Cerebrovascular Accident

The following is an initial examination and evaluation for a patient recently admitted to an inpatient rehab hospital. Use it to help you complete the following 2 SOAP notes.

Initial Examination and Evaluation

Pr: (L) CVA, (R) hemiparesis

Hx: This 67-year-old male was admitted to acute care 08-08-88 due to sudden weakness in his (R) UE & LE and slurred speech. Pt's PMH includes NIDDM, CABG x 2 07-05-85. No other pertinent medical history.

S: *C/o:* Inability to move around like he used to. Weakness in (R) LE & UE

Prior level of function: (I) c̄ all ADL's and gait s̄ assistive device. Active; worked in his woodshop, yard, and garden. Pt. is (R) handed dominant.

Home situation: Lives c̄ wife who is healthy but is a small woman. Lives in 2-level home c̄ 4 steps to enter.

O: *Observation:* Noted 3+ pitting edema in (R) hand and forearm; pt. has tendency to keep (R) UE in dependent position.

Sensation: Pt. displays diminished light touch, deep pressure localization, proprioception & kinesthesia through the (R) UE & LE.

Tone: Pt. displays diminished tone on (R) UE & LE to passive range, diminished patellar reflexes, and absent Achilles reflex on (R)

MMT: (L) UE & LE; 5/5 throughout all musculature (R) UE shoulder flex, ext, abd, MR & LR 2-/5; elbow flex 2+/5, ext 2/5; grip 1/5; (R) LE hip ext, add, IR 3+/5; flex, add, LR 2+/5; knee ext 3-/5, flex 2-/5; ankle df 0/5, pf 1/5.

Mobility: Max (A) scooting ↕ in bed, Mod (A) scooting (R) & (L) in bed; SBA for safety and v/c when rolling to (R); max (A) rolling to (L)

Transfers: Supine ↔ sit Max (A) from (R) side and Mod (A) from (L) side; sit ↔ stand max (A); stand pivot w/c ↔ bed Max (A).

Gait: Not attempted at this time

Balance: Fair static and poor dynamic sitting balance; standing balance very poor.

Endurance: Fair; pt. tolerated 30 minute session requiring 1 minute rest breaks every 5-8 minutes.

A: *PT Dx:* Impaired motor function and muscular performance due to CVA. Prognosis is good for goals as stated. Skilled service needed to help patient improve strength and functional mobility including gait and transfers so that he can return home.

Problem List:

1. Edema in (R) UE

2. Decreased strength in (R) UE & LE

3. Dependent bed mobility

4. Dependent transfers

5 Non-ambulatory

6. Diminished balance

7. Diminished endurance

STG's:

1. Pt. will be able to demonstrate understanding of appropriate positioning for (R) UE.

2. Increase strength (R) UE & LE ½ grade throughout.

3. Pt. will require Mod (A) scooting ↕ in bed, Min (A) scooting (R) & (L) in bed; Mod (A) rolling to (L) and be (I) rolling to (R).

4. Pt. will require Mod (A) for supine ↔ sit from (R), Min (A) supine ↔ sit from (L), Mod (A) for sit ↔ stand and w/c ↔ bed transfers.

5. Pt. will stand $\bar{c}$ Max (A) and quad cane for 1 minute.

6. Pt. will display fair static and fair dynamic sitting balance and fair static standing balance.

7. Pt. will display adequate endurance to tolerate a 30 minute therapy session only needing one 2 minute rest break.

LTG's:

1. Pt. will be (I) in (R) UE self-care.

2. Increase strength (R) UE & LE 1 grade throughout.

3. Pt. will be (I) $\bar{c}$ bed mobility including scooting $\updownarrow$ and $\leftrightarrow$ in bed and rolling to (R) or (L).

4. Pt. will be (I) $\bar{c}$ sit $\leftrightarrow$ stand and w/c $\leftrightarrow$ bed transfers.

5. Pt. will ambulate 20' $\bar{c}$ assistive device as indicated with Mod (A).

6. Pt. will display good static and dynamic sitting balance, fair + static and fair dynamic standing balance.

7. Pt. will display adequate endurance for a 1 hour session of therapy $\bar{c}$ only one 5 minute rest break.

P: PT BID for neuromuscular reeducation, strengthening, mobility training, pre-gait activities, endurance activities, balance training, and education related to positioning and self-care.

Mary Jane, PT

1. You are working with a 67-year-old patient who suffered a (L) CVA. Today the patient states he feels he is getting stronger and is looking forward to his first day-pass to go home with his wife this weekend. The patient's wife states she is concerned about how they will manage in the long run. She says that their son and daughter-in-law are coming in from out of town to help out this weekend. In therapy today, you worked on his bed mobility and transfers. He needed moderate assistance when scooting up and down in bed and scooting to the right. He needed minimal assistance when scooting to the left. He was able to roll to the right without any assistance and was safe with the activity. He required moderate assistance when rolling to the left. The patient still displays significant edema in his right hand and forearm and forgets to use his positioning devices in bed and in the wheelchair. He required minimal assistance when coming up from his left side. He requires minimal assistance when performing a sit to stand transfer and moderate assistance with a stand pivot transfer from the therapy mat into the wheelchair. You educated the patient's wife regarding his need for supervision and constant verbal cues, to perform wheelchair set up, and because he is impulsive and unsafe at times. Review the initial evaluative note so that you can make appropriate comparisons with his initial status. Be sure to include a summary of how is he progressing toward his goals as established by the PT, and write an appropriate plan.

2. One week later, the patient has returned from a weekend pass with his family. The family had considerable difficulty caring for the patient at home, and they feel the home is not set up well for caring for him. The patient is upset at how difficult being at home was. He needs lots of extra encouragement today to participate in therapy. During his therapy session today, the patient requires moderate to maximal assistance with rolling and scooting in bed and for supine to sit transfers when coming up from his right side, and minimal assistance when coming up from his left side. He requires maximal assistance when performing a sit to stand transfer and moderate assistance with a modified stand pivot transfer from the therapy mat into the wheelchair. The patient needs moderate assistance and constant verbal cues to perform set up and is impulsive and a safety risk, today more than usual, due to his bad mood associated with his weekend. In your note, include a summary of how these findings compare with findings from the previous note and the initial evaluative note. Also, briefly comment on the status of his goals and write an appropriate plan.

Lower Extremity Amputation/Prosthetic Devices

The following is an initial examination and evaluation for a patient recently admitted to an inpatient rehab hospital. Use it to help you complete the following 2 SOAP notes.

Initial Examination and Evaluation

Date: January 15, 2005

Pr: 72-year-old male 4 days s/p (R) BKA

S: *History:* Long history of chronic wounds on the (R) foot; recently developed osteomyelitis and gangrene and underwent short transtibial (BK) amputation.

C/C: Phantom pain from the (R) foot, poor mobility, and decreased endurance.

L/S: Pt. is retired coal minor. Lives alone in single-level house, with 2 steps at the entrance. Has never used an assistive device. Has been independent with all ADLs and IADLs prior to admission. PMH includes NIDDM, COPD, PVD, and HTN. Pt. is a non-smoker and non-drinker, although smoked 1 pack per day for 30 years. Quit when he was 50-year-old. Has 1 son living about 2 hours away who can assist on the weekends.

Pt's Goals: Return to independent, active L/S, including driving. Wants to obtain a prosthetic device.

Communication: Pt. communicates goals and needs without difficulty.

O: *AROM:* (B) UEs are WNL; (L) LE is WNL; Right hip flexion 90°, extension 0°, abduction 40°, adduction 10°; knee flexion 90°, extension -10°.

PROM: (R) knee extension -5°.

Strength: (B) UEs and (L) LE are 4/5 throughout; (R) LE not assessed 2° to acuity.

Sensation: (L) LE is intact to light touch, (R) residual limb demonstrates diminished light touch sensation around suture line.

Incision: Horizontal incision line at distal aspect of the residual limb, no tension, complete closure, no drainage.

Pulses: Popliteal artery 2+ bilaterally. Residual limb length is 2″ from tibial tuberosity.

Edema:	(R)	(L)
Knee joint	22 cm	20 cm
2″ below	22.5 cm	19 cm
4″ below	23 cm	18.5 cm

Balance: Not impaired when standing in // bars.

Bed Mobility: (I) c̄ rolling and scooting.

Transfers: Supine ↔ sit with min (A) x 1; sit ↔ stand with min (A) x 1; toilet transfers performed c̄ min (A) x 1.

Gait: Ambulated 10′ x 1 in // bars with CGA x 1 and 25′ c̄ standard walker c̄ min (A) x 1. Balance impaired when ambulating with walker 2° to ↓ weight of (R) limb.

Wheelchair management: Requires max (A) for wheelchair management and can propel ~20′ on level surfaces and then requires a rest break.

Endurance: Unable to ambulate more than 25′ without SOB.

Ther Ex: 20′ of exercises including hip AROM: flexion, extension, abduction, and adduction; knee flexion and extension; hamstring stretching and towel propping.

A: *PT diagnosis:* Impaired motor function, muscle performance, range of motion, gait, locomotion, and balance associated with amputation. Prognosis is good for anticipated goals and outcomes. Patient requiring skilled services for improving functional mobility including gait and transfer training with assistive devices 2° to amputation. Also required for preparing residual limb for prosthesis.

Problem List:

Impairments:

1. Decreased ROM right LE; especially hip extension and knee extension

2. Decreased strength right LE

3. Decreased sensation

4. Edema

5. Incision present

6. Impaired balance with walker

7. Phantom pain

Functional Limitations:

1. Decreased independence with ambulation

2. Decreased independence with transfers

3. At risk for non-healing incision and skin abnormalities

4. Impaired endurance

5. Unable to drive

6. Unable to perform necessary IADLs (grocery shopping, going to bank, etc)

7. Wants to return to active L/S using a prosthetic device

Anticipated Goals and Expected Outcomes:

After 8 weeks pt. will:

1. Demonstrate full A/PROM in the right LE with no contractures—necessary for normal prosthetic ambulation

2. (R) LE strength 4/5 also to allow normal prosthetic ambulation

3. (I) with skin care and monitoring skin with use of prosthesis

4. Demonstrate 100% healing of his incision

5. 50% reduction in c/o phantom pain

6. Ambulate 100' with walker independently

7. Ambulate 150' independently with prosthesis and least restrictive assistive device

8. Transfer in/out of bed (I) and perform sit ↔ stand (I)

9. Obtain driving assessment

10. Participate in a community outing with only min (A) x 1

P: See pt. for 1 hour bid for ~8 weeks to work on the above through active and passive exercise, endurance training, gait and transfer training, pain modulation, balance, and pt. education. The patient is motivated and agrees with the above plan.

Betty Bopp, PT

1. The patient is now 2 weeks s/p right transtibial amputation. He is continuing to complain of phantom pain and sensation from the right foot. It resolves if he "squeezes" his residual limb. You are planning to attend a team conference for him on the following day, so you decide to take some objective measurements. Right AROM is: hip flexion 120°, extension 5°, abduction 40°, adduction 10°; knee flexion 130°, extension -5°. PROM: Right knee extension 0°. Strength: Right LE hip flexion 4/5, extension holds against moderate resistance in side lying position, abduction holds against moderate resistance in side lying position; knee extension holds against minimal resistance in seated position; knee flexion holds against moderate resistance in side lying position. The patient can not lay prone due to pulmonary problems and difficulty breathing when in this position. The incision is healing well. There is no drainage and no signs or symptoms of infection. The incision is moderately adhered to the underlying tissue and hypersensitive to pressure. Residual limb girth is 20 cm at the knee joint, 21 cm 2" below, and 20 cm 4" below. The patient can move and transfer in and out of bed independently to a bedside commode or chair.

He can manage the wheelchair parts with verbal cuing. He propels the wheelchair 50' independently on level surfaces and carpet and then requires a rest. He can ambulate 75' with a standard walker with supervision x 1 and his balance is good. You spent the next 15 minutes on patient education and exercise. You will discuss prosthetic options with the PT and, if appropriate, with the rehab team the following day.

2. The patient is now 7 weeks s/p right transtibial amputation. He is continuing to complain of phantom pain and sensation from the right foot occasionally, but it has decreased by about 75%. He has had a temporary prosthesis for about 2 days. Right AROM is: hip flexion 120°, extension 10°, abduction 40°, adduction 10°; knee flexion 130°, extension 0°. Strength: Right LE hip flexion 4/5, extension holds against moderate resistance in side lying position, abduction holds against moderate resistance in side lying position; knee extension holds against moderate resistance in seated position; knee flexion holds against maximum resistance in side lying position. The incision is not adhered to the underlying tissue and sensitivity has subsided. Residual limb girth is 20 at the knee joint, 19 cm 2" below, and 19 cm 4" below. He is independent with all wheelchair parts and transfer. He propels the wheelchair 500' independently on level surfaces and carpet. He can ambulate 150' with axillary crutches with supervision x 1 and good balance without the prosthesis. You spent the next 30 minutes on prosthetic training. He requires minimal assist to don and doff the socket and secure the supracondylar cuff suspension. He ambulates 50' with the prosthesis on and with axillary crutches with minimal assist for advancing the prosthesis. He is ambulating with an abducted gait on the prosthetic side. You spend 10 minutes educating the patient on skin precautions after removing the prosthesis and 15 minutes on exercises.

Additional considerations:

- Write the "A" and "P" portions of the notes based on available information here and in the evaluative note.
- Write your notes to maximize reimbursement.
- Be specific when documenting your interventions (patient education, coordination, or communication with other disciplines and procedural intervention). What would be appropriate based on the plan of care provided and the patient's status?
- What would corresponding FIM scores be for this patient at the 2 points described above?

Musculoskeletal Trauma

The following is an initial examination and evaluation for a patient recently admitted to an inpatient rehab hospital. Use it to help you complete the following 2 SOAP notes.

Initial Examination and Evaluation

Date: March 1, 2005

Referral from MD: 27-year-old ♂ s/p (L) wrist and ankle fx; Begin gentle wrist and ankle AROM & PROM; May begin using cx c̄ platform for (L) UE. PWB 50% on (L) LE.

S: *HPI:* 4 weeks s/p fall (~25') from a logging truck landing on his (L) side (2/1/04). Pt. sustained fx of the (L) distal radius and ulna and (L) distal tibia and fibular. Pt. underwent ORIF for the wrist and ankle immediately p̄ the injury. He was placed in a SAC for the UE and SLC for the LE. He was NWB on the (L) LE and has been unable to use cx 2° to not being allowed to bear weight on the affected UE. At the time of the fall, the pt. also sustained a mild concussion. He was hospitalized for 5 days following the injury. While hospitalized he received IP PT to learn how to negotiate his w/c and perform transfers. Both casts were removed yesterday, and his ankle was placed in a removable splint. Reports taking ibuprofen PRN for pain.

C/C: Pain and stiffness in (L) UE & LE c̄ ↓ functional use of (B). Doesn't like using w/c for mobility. Unable to work. Requiring assist c̄ self-care activities and home management.

L/S: RHD; Lives c̄ wife and 2 small children in single level home c̄ 2 steps @ entrance c̄ HR on the (R). Prior to injury pt. was employed as a construction worker. He has been off work since the DOI. Pt. is unable to drive and is relying on his wife & mother for transportation. No significant PMH or hx of fx. Reports being a non-smoker and non-drinker. Family hx is (+) for OA.

Pt's Goals: Return to previous level of function and RTW ASAP. Learn to ambulate with cx.

O: *AROM:* (R) UE & LE WNL; (L) shoulder, elbow, & hip WNL

(L) wrist:	AROM	PROM
Flexion	20°	25°
Extension	10°	15°
UD	10°	15°
RD	15°	15°
Supination	30°	35°
Pronation	40°	45°

(L) hand: Pt. can perform a full fist but it is difficult 2° to edema. Thumb IP, MCP, and CMC AROM is WNL

(L) knee:	0-100°	0-110°

(L) ankle:		
DF	-10°	-5°
PF	20°	25°
Inv	5°	5°
Ev	0°	5°

Strength: (R) UE & LE 5/5; (L) shoulder and hip 4/5; (L) elbow, wrist, knee, & ankle deferred 2° to acuity

Girth: wrist figure 8 (R): 36 cm (L): 37.2 cm; ankle figure 8 (R): 42 cm (L): 44.1 cm

Sensation: (L) wrist and ankle intact to light touch & = when compared to (R)

Circulation: 2+ at radial & dorsal pedal arteries on the (L)

Special Tests: N/A @ this time 2° to acuity

Gait: Unable to ambulate at this time

Transfers: (I) bed ↔ chair, chair ↔ toilet, sit ↔ stand all NWB on (L) LE

Bed Mobility: (I) all areas

Tx & HEP: AROM & PROM for (L) wrist for flexion, extension, & supination and for (L) ankle DF and PF, used opposite foot for self PROM of ankle; performed AROM for all digits and thumb; initiated compression glove for edema to be worn n.s.; instructed pt. in elevation and compression wrapping for ankle and wrist; instructed pt. in use of cx with platform for (L) UE PWB 50% (L) using step to gait pattern. Pt. required CGA x 1 for balance. The pt. performed all ex. (I) and verbalized understanding of all precautions.

A: *PT Diagnosis:* 27-year-old RHD ♂, 4 wks s/p fall. Impaired mobility, muscle performance, and range of motion associated with fx to the (L) wrist & ankle. Now c̄ ↓ AROM, PROM, and strength. Inability to ambulate, perform self-care or home management tasks without assist. Unable to work @ this time. Skilled services necessary to instruct pt. in appropriate ROM ex., use of AD & progress gait as ordered. Also will require strengthening and functional mobility retraining to prepare for return to normal L/S and RTW. Pt. able to communicate without limitations and demonstrates excellent motivation and good potential for full recovery. No co-morbidities that could affect outcome identified at this time.

Anticipated Goals and Expected Outcomes:

At the end of 2 weeks, the pt. will:

1. Increase AROM 10-15° for the wrist, forearm, and ankle

2. Decrease edema by .5 cm for the wrist and ankle

3. Ambulate c̄ cx c̄ (L) UE platform PWB (L) LE (I)

4. Perform all self-care (I)

5. Perform a full fist s̄ limitations

At the end of 16 weeks (d/c), the pt. will:

1. Have normal AROM of the wrist, forearm, and ankle (90-100% of opposite)

2. Grip and pinch strength will be 80-100% of (R)

3. Be (I) c̄ all self-care & home management tasks

4. Ambulate (I) on all surfaces s̄ use of AD

5. ↑↓ flight of stairs (I) s̄ AD

6. Drive s̄ restrictions

7. RTW @ previous level of employment

P: See pt. 3x/wk for next 3-4 mos. to work on AROM & PROM of the wrist and ankle; general LE ex. for the hip, knee, shoulder, and elbow; gait training; functional mobility; & strengthening when appropriate. Will progress pt. as tolerated & according to MD orders. Pt. is in agreement c̄ the above stated plan.

John Smith, PT

1.   The patient is now 6 weeks s/p fall. He is reporting improvement in his ability to perform self-care, achieve a full fist, and ambulate. He thinks the exercises are helping to improve all of these activities. He is seeing the doctor today and is hoping to be able to discontinue the use of the crutches. You take the following AROM measurements for the left wrist: flexion 50°, extension35°, supination 50°, pronation 60°. Left knee 0-135°, left ankle -10° from neutral DF, and has 45° of PF. He has 10° of inversion and 2° of eversion. He can perform all transfers independently and ambulates 100′ independently PWB on the left LE with cx with a left platform. Wrist figure 8 is 36.7 cm on the left, and ankle figure 8 is 43.4 on the left. You are still not performing strength assessment due to fractures. You spend 45 minutes working on exercises to increase range of motion for the ankle and wrist and reviewing his home exercises.

2.   The patient is now 9 weeks s/p fall. He is reporting independence with self-care, ambulation, and driving. He thinks the exercises are helping to improve all of these activities and improve strength necessary for returning to work. He is ambulating full weight bearing on the left, without use of crutches. You take the following AROM measurements for the left wrist: flexion 80°, extension 65°, supination 75°, pronation 80°. Left knee 0-140°, left ankle 0° (neutral) DF, and has 50° of PF. He has 15° of inversion and 5° of eversion. He can ambulate for unlimited distances around the house and the community. He does have some mild swelling after ambulating distances greater than 400-500′. Wrist figure 8 is 36 cm on the left, and ankle figure 8 is 43 on the left. Grip strength measured via JAMAR #2 was 120 pounds on the right and 62 pounds on the left. You spend 45 minutes working on exercises to increase range of motion for the ankle and wrist and reviewing his home exercises.

For these notes, you will need to come up with "A" and "P" based on information provided here and in the evaluation on the previous page. Also, provide more detail of your intervention(s), ie, specific exercises to accomplish goals, education, and communication with other providers.

Pediatrics/Orthotic Devices

The following is an initial examination and evaluation for a patient recently referred to outpatient PT. Use it to help you complete the following 2 SOAP notes.

Pr: 5-year-old female with L3 level myelomeningocele, referred to PT for transfer training, gait training, and orthotic management.

S: *Hx:* Myelomeningocele present at birth. Immediate surgery to repair. Resultant L3 incomplete paralysis. No history of hydrocephalus or seizure d/o.

C/C: Impaired ability to transfer independently; decreased independence with ambulation.

L/S: Lives with both parents who are very supportive. Attends kindergarten at a local, public elementary school.

Pt. and Parents' Goals: Increase independence with transfers, participate in circle time on the floor without having to be transferred by the teacher, ambulate household distances and distances at school independently, manage wheelchair independently.

Cognition/Communication: Able to communicate without difficulty and express goals of therapy. At grade level for all school-related cognitive tasks per parental report.

O: *AROM:* (B) UEs are WNL; LEs: hip flexion 120°, extension 0°, abduction 40°, adduction 10°; knee flexion 0°, extension 0°.

PROM: Bilateral knees 0°-135°; ankles DF 20° and PF 50°.

Strength: (B) UEs 4/5 throughout; LEs: Right hip flexion 3+/5, extension 3/5, abduction 3/5, adduction 3+/5; knee extension 3/5; left hip flexion 4/5, extension 3+/5, abduction 3+/5, adduction 4/5; knee extension 3+/5. All others are 0/5.

Sensation: Left: Normal sensation in L1, 2, and 3 dermatomes; diminished in L4 and L5, absent in S1; Right: Normal sensation in L1 and 2; diminished in L3, L4, and L5, absent in S1.

Posture: Normal spinal alignment and absence of joint contractures or abnormal posture of feet and ankles.

Spasticity: Mild in (B) hip adductors, IR, and heel cords right > left.

Bowel/bladder: Incontinent in bowel and bladder control but is independently managed by parents and teacher.

Skin Condition: No impairments other than small area on right navicular from pressure from orthotic device.

Anthropometrics: Normal body weight for height.

Balance: Not impaired when standing in // bars with (B) UE support.

Bed Mobility: Independent rolling and scooting.

Transfers: Supine ↔ long and short sit independently; sit ↔ stand with minimal assist x 1 using lofstrand cx and KAFOs; w/c ↔ floor with maximal assist x 1.

Floor mobility: Independent in floor mobility for short distances using commando crawling.

Wheelchair Management/Mobility: Independent with mobility on level even surfaces for 50-60'; Requires min assist for managing parts including leg rests and arm rests.

Gait: Ambulated 10' x 1 with minimal assist x 1 using step to gait with knees locked at 0° in KAFOs. Balance impaired when ambulating with lofstrands 2° to decreased proprioception and kinesthetic awareness of (B) LEs.

Endurance: Unable to ambulate more than 10' without shortness of breath.

Orthotic devices: Dependent in donning and doffing.

A: *PT Diagnosis:* Impaired motor function and sensory integrity associated with non-progressive disorder of the CNS. Prognosis for anticipated goals and outcomes is good. Skilled service needed to educate patient on appropriate ways to transfer and to increase endurance and strength to allow increased independence with gait and transfers.

Impairments:

1. (B) LE weakness

2. Flaccid ankles

3. Impaired proprioception and kinesthetic awareness during gait

4. Impaired sensation

5. Mild spasticity

6. Impaired endurance

Functional Limitations:

1. Decreased ability to transfer from wheelchair to floor

2. Decreased sit ↔ stand

3. Decreased independence with gait

4. Decreased distance and balance during gait

5. Unable to ascend and descend stairs

6. Requiring assist for managing wheelchair parts

7. Requiring assist to manage orthotic devices

Anticipated goals and expected outcomes:

At the end of 8 weeks, the pt. will:

1. Transfer w/c ↔ floor with minimal assist x 1

2. Perform sit ↔ stand independently

3. Manage wheelchair leg rests and arm rests independently

4. Propel w/c 500' independently

5. Ambulate 100' with KAFOs and bilateral lofstrand cx with close supervision

6. Ascend and descend 3 stairs with minimal assist

7. Don and doff the KAFOs with minimal assist

P: See pt. 2 to 3 x per week to work on the above plan and goals. Will require strengthening, endurance, balance, and gait training to meet above goals. Pt. and parents are in agreement with above plan.

1. It is now the patient's fourth PT visit, and you have been working with this patient for the last 2 visits. She is very motivated and happy to come to therapy. She is very cooperative, and her parents are very supportive and follow through with all instructions as assigned. She demonstrates the ability to transfer from the wheelchair to the floor with minimal assist and verbal cuing. She requires moderate assist to transfer from the floor to the wheelchair. Her UE strength is good via MMT, but she can not lift her own body weight at this point. She performs sit ↔ stand with contact guard assist with KAFOs and lofstrand cx. She can ambulate 40' with minimal assist of 1 with the braces and cx. Still demonstrating impaired dynamic balance. You worked with her for 30 minutes performing UE and LE strengthening and dynamic balance exercises and for an additional 15 minutes on gait training.

2. The patient has been participating in PT for 1 month, you have seen her at every visit with the exceptions of the initial evaluation and during a reevaluation which took place ~ 1 to 2 weeks ago. She is still very cooperative and motivated. She received new KAFOs from the orthotist today. They have a manual locking mechanism at the knee and are rigid at the ankles. Inspection of the devices reveals no problems with hardware, and all edges and rivets are smooth and straps are well-secured. The skin is free from breakdown before donning the devices. The patient requires moderate assist to don the orthotic devices and to engage the knee lock. She ambulated in // bars 10′ using an open-hand technique with minimal assist of 1 and then used her lofstrands using a step to gait pattern also requiring minimal assist. After gait training (lasted ~20 minutes) the patient required moderate assist to doff the orthotic devices. Patient and parent were educated on skin inspection. There was a small area on the right navicular that was red after removing the device on the right. You provided education on monitoring the redness. Leaving the braces off, you performed 30 minutes of exercises for the UEs and LEs and dynamic balance activities.

Additional considerations:

- Write the "A" and "P" portions of the notes based on information available here and in the evaluative notes.
- Write your notes to maximize reimbursement.
- Be specific when documenting your interventions (patient education, coordination or communication with other disciplines, and procedural intervention). What would be appropriate based on the plan of care provided and the patient's status?

Glossary

abuse—Billing for items that are not covered or misusing billing codes. Usually a result of an error or lack of knowledge of proper code(s) or coding procedure(s).

activity limitation—Difficulties or limitations encountered by an individual who is attempting to complete a task or carry out an activity.

advance beneficiary notice (ABN)—A notification that a health care provider asks a Medicare beneficiary to sign when providing a service that may not be covered by Medicare. In signing the ABN, the Medicare beneficiary agrees to pay for the service if it is not covered by Medicare (see also notice of exclusion of Medicare benefits).

carrier—A privately run insurance company that contracts with the government to pay bills for Medicare Part B. Carriers are determined by geographic region and can be found at http://www.cms.hhs.gov/contacts/incardir.asp #4.

case-mix group—Categorization or grouping of patients in hospitals, or other facilities, according to common characteristics such diagnosis, disease, and functional status.

Centers for Medicare and Medicaid Services (CMS)—A federal government agency that administers Medicare and works with state governments to administer Medicaid and State Children's Health Insurance Programs (SCHIP). CMS is housed within the Department of Health and Human Services (www.cms.hhs.gov).

co-morbidity (or co-morbidities)—Aspect(s) of the patient's past medical history that affect(s) his or her current episode of care; or, a previous or current medical condition that has the potential to hinder progress in physical therapy.

diagnosis—A medical diagnosis assigned by a physician identifies the injury, illness, or disease, usually at the cellular, organ, or system level. A diagnosis assigned by a physical therapist identifies the impact of the patient's medical condition and impairments on movement and function.

diagnosis-related group (DRG)—A categorization system used to group patients according to diagnosis, type of treatment, age, and other relevant criteria. DRGs are used as part of the inpatient prospective payment system.

disablement—The consequences of disease as they pertain to the relationship between body structures, the ability to carry out tasks, and the capability to function within society.

disability—The inability or limitation in performing socially defined roles and tasks that would normally be expected of an individual within a given culture or environment.

durable medical equipment (DME)—Medical equipment that has been prescribed by a health care provider that is either purchased or rented by a patient, to be used in the patient's home. Examples include hospital beds, walkers, canes, wheelchairs, and oxygen.

evaluation—An assessment of the patient's condition based on data collected during the physical therapist's examination. It includes consideration of the chronicity, severity, complexity, and extent of impairments, functional limitations, and disabilities.

evidence-based practice—Using the best evidence available (research reports, case studies, textbooks, etc), along with clinical experience, to make patient-care decisions.

examination—A collection of tests and measurements, including questions to determine medical history, current complaints, lifestyle, and physical therapy goals. The examination data is used to identify pertinent physical therapy problems, co-morbidities, rehabilitation potential; to determine expected outcomes; and to develop a plan of care that includes appropriate interventions, consultation with other health care providers, and patient education.

fiscal intermediary (*also known as* intermediary)—A privately run insurance company that contracts with the government to pay bills for Medicare Part A and some Medicare Part B. Fiscal intermediaries are determined by geographic region and can be found at http://www.cms.hhs.gov/contacts/incardir.asp#4.

fraud—Billing an insurance company, Medicare, or other third-party payer for services that were not provided; or, billing for an item or service that has higher reimbursement than the service or item actually provided.

functional independence measure (FIM)—A standardized multidisciplinary evaluation tool often used to score the patient's performance in self-care, bowel and bladder management, transfers, gait and/or wheelchair mobility, communication, and cognition. Patients are scored 1-7 (1 equal to total assist and 7 equal to independent) according to the level of assist they require to complete the task.

functional limitation—An abnormality or limitation, caused by a pathology and/or impairment(s), that affects an individual's ability to carry out a meaningful action, task, or activity.

health care clearinghouse—An entity associated with a health care provider or third-party payer that provides services such as billing, database management, transcription, information technology, etc. The health care clearinghouse has access to patient information but is not involved in patient care.

homebound—Status given to a patient who is unable to leave his home, or when leaving requires significantly taxing efforts. Short infrequent trips, such as medical appointments and religious services, are permitted when a patient has been declared "homebound."

home health care—Skilled nursing or rehabilitative care provided in a patient's home. Home care services can be provided when a patient is declared "homebound."

impairment—A deviation or loss in a body function or structure.

incident report—A report filed in the event of an "incident" that could likely result in a lawsuit. Used to document errors and departures from normal procedures that result in adverse outcomes, procedural breakdowns, and catastrophic events. These reports are completed by the individual involved in the incident, and they are filed with the risk management department.

informed consent—Consent, to a treatment(s) or service(s), given by a patient after being informed of risks, benefits, alternatives, and consequences of no treatment at all.

inpatient rehabilitation facility (IRF)—A hospital or unit, within a larger facility (eg, acute-care hospital), that provides intense rehabilitative services to patients. The majority of patients admitted to an IRF have been diagnosed with one of 13 qualifying medical conditions that have been established by Medicare. Examples are stroke, spinal cord injury, brain injury, amputation, hip fracture, burn, neurological disorder, and knee or hip replacement. More information and the list of qualifying diagnoses can be found at http://www.cms.hhs.gov/medlearn/matters/mmarticles/2004/MM3334.pdf.

maintenance—Services that can be provided by a non-licensed individual, including the patient himself, a family member, or a caregiver who has had some training from a skilled professional. Maintenance services are not reimbursed by Medicare or many other third-party payers.

malpractice—A bad or unskillful act performed by a physician or other professional provider that injures or causes harm to a patient or client; the failure of an individual or group to follow the accepted standards that have been set forth by their respective profession(s); includes willful negligence and ignorant malpractice.

managed care—A type of health care in which an insurance company (or third-party payer) maintains some control over costs and utilization of services and/or benefits.

Medicaid—A joint federal and state program that helps with medical costs for individuals with low incomes and limited resources.

medical necessity—As defined by Centers for Medicare & Medicaid Services, medical necessity is a procedure or intervention that is appropriate and needed for the diagnosis or treatment of a medical condition; is provided for the diagnosis, direct care, and treatment of a medical condition; meets the standards of good medical practice in the local area; *and* is not mainly for the convenience of the patient or health care provider.

Medicare—The federal health insurance program for individuals: (1) 65 years of age and older who are receiving or eligible for social security retirement benefits; (2) younger than 65 with certain disabilities that meet the Social Security Act's disability requirements; and (3) with end-stage renal disease.

notice of exclusion of Medicare benefits (NEMB)—A notification that a health care provider asks a Medicare beneficiary to sign when providing a service that is not covered by Medicare. In signing the NEMB, the Medicare beneficiary agrees to pay for the service not covered by Medicare (*see also* advance beneficiary notice).

outcome—The end result of patient-client management. Could also be the end result of an episode of care.

participation restrictions—Problems an individual faces while involved in life situations.

pathology—Interruption or interference with the body's normal processes and simultaneous body efforts to heal itself or regain a normal state. Often known as the actual disease, or medical diagnosis.

primary care provider (PCP)—A physician responsible for a patient's point-of-entry into the health care system. Some insurance companies require the PCP to be the patient's family physician. The PCP can also be a general practitioner, internal medicine specialist, or, in some cases, an obstetrician/gynecologist.

prognosis—Includes the anticipated goals, the expected frequency and duration of services, the interventions to be used, the expected outcomes, and the ultimate plan for discharge.

prospective payment system (PPS)—Medicare reimbursement provided to facilities (ie, hospitals and skilled nursing facilities) that is predetermined, or fixed, based on the patient's diagnosis and/or complexity.

protected health information—Individually identifiable information referring to an individual's medical history; previous, current, and future medical care; and billing and payment information. Also known as individually identifiable health information. Includes information that could potentially allow identification of the individual, ie, address, telephone and fax number, birth date, admission and discharge dates, voice recordings.

reimbursement—Payment made to a health care provider from an insurance company, or other third-party payer, after being billed for a service provided to a patient.

secondary insurance—Additional or supplemental insurance carried by a patient. The secondary will typically cover additional costs not covered by the individual's primary insurance.

skilled care—A type of health care given when a patient needs management, observation, or evaluation by trained nurses or rehabilitation staff; also includes care that requires the unique judgment and skill of a trained individual for both safety and effectiveness.

skilled nursing facility (SNF)—A free-standing facility, or facility within a hospital, nursing home, or rehabilitation center, that provides skilled medical, nursing, or rehabilitative services to patients. Examples of skilled services include intravenous injections, oxygen, feeding tubes, wound care, and rehabilitation (http://www.cms.hhs.gov/manuals/cmstoc.asp).

state practice act—A state's regulation of licensed professionals. Usually defines the educational (and continuing education) requirements, scope of practice, acceptable service delivery, and licensure requirements.

third-party payer—The insurance company, or other health benefit plan sponsor, that pays for medical services provided to a patient. The patient and the health care provider are considered the 2 primary parties.

utilization review—Examination of medical necessity, economic appropriateness, and quality of care provided to patients by a health care provider. Usually conducted by a managed care organization to determine need for initiation or continuation of health care service.

Appendix A: Abbreviations and Symbols

This list provides many of the abbreviations and symbols used in medical charts and in physical therapy records. Because documentation styles can vary, you should check with your facility regarding abbreviations and symbols that are "approved" for use. Also, note that some abbreviations have more than one meaning. Be sure to understand the context in which each abbreviation is used. *Lists are alphabetized by the abbreviation. However, in some cases where the abbreviation and its meaning do not begin with the same letter, the pair is listed under the abbreviation as well as under the meaning (ie, bid, or twice daily, is listed under "B" for bid and under "T" for twice daily).*

ABBREVIATIONS

A: or "A"	assessment
AAROM	active assistive range of motion
Ab	antibody
abd	abduction
ABG(s)	arterial blood gas(es)
ac	before meals
ACE	angiotensin-converting enzyme
Ach	acetylcholine
ACL	anterior cruciate ligament
AD	assistive device; Alzheimer's disease
ADA	Americans with Disabilities Act
add	adduction
ADL	activities of daily living
ad lib	as desired
ADM	abductor digiti minimi
AE	above elbow
AFB	acid-fast bacilli
AFO	ankle foot orthosis
AGA	appropriate for gestational age
AIDS	acquired immunodeficiency syndrome
AK	above knee
AKA	above knee amputation
ALL	acute lymphoblastic leukemia
ALS	amyotrophic lateral sclerosis
am	before noon
AMA	against medical advice
AMB	ambulatory
AML	acute myeloblastic leukemia
ANOVA	analysis of variance
AP	ankle pump; anterior-posterior
APB	abductor pollicus brevis
APL	abductor pollicus longus
ARDS	adult (acute) respiratory distress syndrome
AROM	active range of motion
ASA	aspirin
ASAP	as soon as possible
ASHD	arteriosclerotic heart disease
ATF	anterior talofibular
AV	atriovenous
n.s.	at bedtime
pc	after meals
pm	after noon
PRN	as needed

BBB	blood brain barrier	d/c	discharge or discontinue
BE	below elbow	DC	doctor of chiropractic; chiropractor
bid	twice daily	DF	dorsiflexion
BK	below knee	DI	dorsal interossei
BKA	below knee amputation	DIP	distal interphalangeal
BLE or (B)LE	bilateral lower extremities	DM	diabetes mellitus
BM	bowel movement	DME	durable medical equipment
BMD	bone mineral density	DMERC	durable medical equipment regional carrier
BMI	body mass index	DO	doctor of osteopath
BP	blood pressure	DOI	date of injury
BPH	benign prostatic hypertrophy	DRG	diagnosis-related group
BPM or bpm	beats per minute	DRUJ	distal radioulnar joint
BRP	bathroom privileges	DTR	deep tendon reflex
BSA	body surface area	DVT	deep vein thrombosis
BUN	blood urea nitrogen	dx	diagnosis
po	by mouth		
		ea.	each
Ca	calcium	ECF	extracellular fluid
CA	cancer	ECRB	extensor carpi radialis brevis
CABG	coronary artery bypass graft	ECRL	extensor carpi radialis longus
CAD	coronary artery disease	ECU	extensor carpi ulnaris
CAT	computerized axial tomography	EDC	extensor digitorum communis
CBC	complete blood count	EDM	extensor digiti minimi
c/c or C/C	chief complaint	EEG	electroencephalogram
cc or cm3	cubic centimeter	EENT	eyes, ears, nose, and throat
CCU	critical (or coronary) care unit	EIP	extensor indicis proprius
CDC	Center for Disease Control	EKG, ECG	electrocardiogram
CF	calcaneofibular	EMG	electromyogram
CF	cystic fibrosis	EMS	emergency medical services
CGA	contact guard assist	ENG	electronystagmograph
CHI	closed head injury	EO	elbow orthosis
CHO	carbohydrate	EPB	extensor pollicus brevis
Cl	chlorine	EPL	extensor pollicus longus
cm	centimeter	ERV	expiratory reserve volume
CMC	carpometacarpal	ESR	erythrocyte sedimentation rate
CMS	Center for Medicare and Medicaid Services	ESRD	end-stage renal disease
CMV	cytomegalovirus	EtOH or ETOH	ethyl alcohol
CNS	central nervous system	ev, ever	eversion
c/o	complains of	ex.	exercise
COPD	chronic obstructive pulmonary disease	q	every
CORF	comprehensive outpatient rehabilitation facility	q2h	every two hours
		q3h	every three hours
COTA	certified occupational therapist assistant	q4h	every four hours
CP	cerebral palsy	q8h	every eight hours
CPAP	continuous positive airway pressure	qam	every morning
CPM	continuous passive motion	qh	every hour
CPR	cardiopulmonary resuscitation	qod	every other day
C & S	culture and sensitivity		
CSF	cerebrospinal fluid		
CT	computed tomography	F or 3/5	fair (manual muscle test)
CV	cardiovascular	FBS	fasting blood sugar
CVA	cerebrovascular accident	FCR	flexor carpi radialis
CWP	cold whirlpool	FCU	flexor carpi ulnaris
cx	cancel; crutches	FDA	Food and Drug Administration

FDM	flexor digiti minimi
FDP	flexor digitorum profundus
FDS	flexor digitorum superficialis
FES	functional electrical stimulation
FEV	forced expiratory volume
FHR	fetal heart rate
fl	fluid
FM	Fibromyalgia Syndrome
FO	foot orthosis
FPB	flexor pollicus brevis
FPL	flexor pollicus longus
FRC	functional residual capacity
FTSG	full thickness skin graft
FUO	fever of unknown origin
FVC	forced vital capacity
FWB	full weight bearing
FWW	front wheeled walker
fx	fracture
qid	four times a day
G or 4/5	good (manual muscle test)
g	gram
GA	gestational age
GERD	gastroesophageal reflux disease
GH	glenohumeral
GI	gastrointestinal
GS	gluteal sets
GTT	glucose tolerance test
H₂O	water
h or hr	hour
HAV	hepatitis A virus; hallux abductovalgus
Hb	hemoglobin
HBV	hepatitis B virus
HCFA	Health Care Financing Administration
HCPCS	health care common procedure coding system
Hct	hematocrit
HCV	hepatitis C virus
HDL	high-density lipoprotein
HEP	home exercise program
H & H	hemoglobin and hematocrit
HHA	home health agency
HIV	human immunodeficiency virus
HMO	health maintenance organization
HNP	herniated nucleus pulposus
h/o	history of
HO	hand orthosis
HO	hip orthosis
HOB	head of bed
H & P	history and physical
HP	hot pack
HPI	history of present illness
HR	hand rail; heart rate
HRT	hormone replacement therapy
HTN	hypertension

hx	history
Hz	hertz
IADL	instrumental activities of daily living
IC	inspiratory capacity
ICD	International Classification of Disease
ICF	intracellular fluid; International Classification of Functioning, Disability, and Health
ICIDH	International Classification of Impairments, Disabilities, and Handicaps
ICP	intracranial pressure
ICU	intensive care unit
I & D	incision and drainage
IDDM	insulin-dependent diabetes mellitus
IDEA	Individuals with Disabilities in Education Act
Ig	immunoglobulin
IM	intramuscular
INH	isoniazid
inv	inversion
I & O	intake and output
IP	inpatient; interphalangeal
IPPS	inpatient prospective payment system
IRV	inspiratory reserve volume
IV	intravenous
stat	immediately
K	potassium
KAFO	knee ankle foot orthosis
kg	kilogram
(L)	left
L	liter
LAC	long arm cast
LAQ	long arc quadriceps exercise
LCL	lateral collateral ligament
LDL	low-density lipoprotein
LE	lower extremity
LHD	left hand dominant
LLC	long leg cast
LMN	lower motor neuron
LMRP	local medical review policies
LP	lumbar puncture
L/S, l/s	lifestyle
LT	lunotriquetrial
LTFG	long term functional goal
LTG	long term goal
LTM	long term memory
m	meter
m.	muscle
MCL	medial collateral ligament
MCP	metacarpophalangeal
MD	Muscular Dystrophy; medical doctor/physician
MED(S)	medicines, medications
MG	Myasthenia Gravis
MHz	megahertz

MI	myocardial infarction
MID	multi-infarct dementia
mm	millimeter
mm Hg	millimeters of mercury
MMT	manual muscle test
MOI	mechanism of injury
mos	months
MRI	magnetic resonance image
MRSA	methicillin-resistant Staphylococcus aureus
MS	Multiple Sclerosis
MTP	metatarsophalangeal
mV	millivolt
MVA	motor vehicle accident
N or 5/5	normal (manual muscle test)
N	newton
n.	nerve
Na	sodium
N/A	not applicable
NBQC	narrow base quad cane
NDT	neurodevelopmental treatment
NICU	neonatal intensive care unit
NIDDM	non-insulin dependent diabetes mellitus
NIH	National Institutes of Health
NMES	neuromuscular electrical stimulation
NPO	nothing by mouth
n.s.	at bedtime
NSAID(S)	non-steroidal anti-inflammatory drug(s)
NT	not tested
n & v	nausea and vomiting
NWB	non-weight bearing
O: or "O"	objective
O2 or O_2	oxygen
OA	osteoarthritis
OASIS	outcome & assessment information set
OB/GYN	obstetrics and gynecology
OBS	organic brain syndrome
OCD	obsessive compulsive disorder
ODM	opponens digitit minimi
OI	Osteogenesis Imperfecta
OOB	out of bed
OP	opponens pollicus; outpatient
OR	operating room
ORIF	open reduction internal fixation
OSHA	Occupational Safety & Health Administration
OT	occupational therapist
OTC	over-the-counter (ie, drugs)
OTR/L	occupational therapist registered and licensed
oz	ounce

SaO_2	oxygen saturation
P or 2/5	poor (manual muscle test)
P: or "P"	plan
p	probability of success
p!	pain
PA	posterior-anterior
PA-C	physician assistant
pc	after meals
PCA	patient-controlled anesthesia
PCL	posterior cruciate ligament
PD	Parkinson's disease
PDR	Physicians' Desk Reference
PE	pulmonary embolism
PEG	percutaneous endoscopic gastrostomy (tube)
PERRLA	pupils equal, round (regular), reactive to light, and accommodating
PET	positron emission tomography
PF	plantarflexion
PFT	pulmonary function test
PI	palmar interossei
PIP	proximal interphalangeal
PL	palmaris longus
pm	after noon
PMH	past (or previous) medical history
PNF	proprioceptive neuromuscular facilitation
PNS	peripheral nervous system
po	by mouth
POMR	problem-oriented medical record
post-op	post-operative
PPO	preferred provider organization
PPS	prospective payment system
PQ	pronator quadratus
PRN	as needed
PROM	passive range of motion
PRUJ	proximal radioulnar joint
PT	physical therapist; pronator teres; prothrombin time
pt. or Pt.	patient
PTA	physical therapist assistant; prior to admission
PTCA	percutaneous transluminal coronary angioplasty
PTF	posterior talofibular
PTT	partial thromboplastin time
PVD	peripheral vascular disease
PWB	partial weight bearing (usually 50% unless otherwise indicated; may need to check with physician to clarify)
K	Potassium
MD	physician
Rx	prescription
q	every
q2h	every two hours
q3h	every three hours

q4h	every four hours	STSG	split thickness skin graft
q8h	every eight hours	Na	sodium
qam	every morning		
qh	every hour	T or 1/5	trace (manual muscle test)
qid	four times a day	T	temperature
qod	every other day	TA	therapeutic activity
QS	quad set/quadriceps set	TB	tuberculosis
		TBI	traumatic brain injury
® or (R)	right	tbsp or T	tablespoon
RA	rheumatoid arthritis	TFCC	triangular fibrocartilagenous complex
RBC	red blood cell	THA	total hip arthroplasy
RC	radiocarpal	THR	total hip replacement
RCL	radial collateral ligament	TIA	transient ischemic attack
RD	radial deviation	tid	three times a day
RDS	respiratory distress syndrome	TKA	total knee arthroplasy
reps	repetitions	TKE	terminal knee extension
RGO	reciprocating gait orthosis	TKR	total knee replacement
RHD	right hand dominant	TMJ	tempromandibular joint
r/o; R/O	rule out	TP	therapeutic procedure
ROM	range of motion	TPN	total parenteral nutrition
ROS	review of systems	tsp or t	teaspoon
RPE	rate of perceived exertion	TTP	tender to palpation
RR	respiratory rate	TTWB	toe touch weight bearing
r/s	reschedule	TV	tidal volume
RT	respiratory therapy	tx	traction or treatment
RTC	return to clinic	bid	twice daily
RTW	return to work		
RV	residual volume	UCL	ulnar collateral ligament
Rx	prescription	UD	ulnar deviation
		UE	upper extremity
S: or "S"	subjective	UMN	upper motor neuron
s or SVN	supervision	US	ultrasound
SAC	short arm cast	UTI	urinary tract infection
SaO$_2$	oxygen saturation	UV	ultraviolet
SAQ	short arc quadriceps exercise		
SBA	stand by assist	V	volt
SCI	spinal cord injury		
SIDS	sudden infant death syndrome	W	watt
SL	Scapholunate; side lying	WBAT	weight bearing as tolerated
SLC	short leg cast	WBC	white blood cell
SLE	systemic lupus erythmatosus	WBQC	wide base quad cane
SLP	speech language pathologist	w/c	wheelchair
SLR	straight leg raise	w/cm^2	watts per centimeters squared
SMA	Spinal Muscular Atrophy	WFL	within functional limits
SO	shoulder orthosis	WHFO	wrist hand finger orthosis
SOB	shortness of breath	WHO	wrist hand orthosis; World Health Organization
s/p	status post		
SPT	student physical therapist	wk	week
SPTA	student physical therapist assistant	WNL	within normal limits
ST	scapulothoracic	WP	whirlpool
stat	immediately	WWP	warm whirlpool
STG	short term goal	H$_2$O	water
STM	short-term memory		
		y.o.	year old

COMMON SYMBOLS

about	~
after	$\bar{p}$
ascend or increase	↑
assist (min, mod, max assist)	(a) or (A)
at	@
before	$\bar{a}$
both or bilateral	(B) or Ⓑ
degrees	°
degrees Celsius	°C
degrees Fahrenheit	°F
dependent	(D)
descend or decrease	↓
equal, equal to	(=)
extension	/
female	♀
flexion	✓
for, except	x
greater than, greater than or equal to	>, ≥
hour, foot	'
inch, minute	"
independent	(I)
left	(L) or Ⓛ
less than, less than or equal to	<, ≤
male	♂
micron	μ
negative	(-) or ⊝
not equal to, unequal	≠
number of individuals assisting (one, two)	x1, x2
parallel (as in parallel bars)	// (// bars)
per	/
positive	(+) or ⊕
possible, question, suggestive	?
pounds	# or lbs.
primary	1°
right	(R) or Ⓡ
sample mean	$\bar{x}$
secondary, secondary to	2°, 2° to
times (as in 3 times per day)	x (3x/day)
up and down or ascend and descend	↑↓
with	$\bar{c}$
without	$\bar{s}$

Appendix B:
Sample Forms and Templates

Jeff Erickson, MS, PT, ATC, SCS, CSCS

GENERAL PHYSICAL THERAPY EVALUATION FORM

Anytown Physical Therapy and Rehabilitation
Physical Therapy Examination and Evaluation Form

Patient's Name:_____ Age:_____ Date:_____

Physician:_____ Diagnosis:_____

Reason for Referral:_____

Injured Side: Right   Left   Hand Dominance: Right   Left

History:

HPI:_____

_____

_____

_____

History of similar problem: ❏ No   ❏ Yes_____

C/C:_____

Pain Scale (0-10):_____

Activities that increase pain:_____

Activities that decrease pain:_____

Previous treatment:_____

Diagnostic Testing/Imaging:_____

Numbness/Tingling: ❏ No   ❏ Yes_____

Temperature changes: ❏ No   ❏ Yes_____

Orthotic/prosthetic devices: ❏ No   ❏ Yes_____

L/S:

Lives with:_____

Home environment:_____

Employment/Work/School Status:_____

Occupation:_____

PMH:_____

Family Medical History:_____

Current medication(s): _____

Social/Health Habits (Smoking/Drinking Alcohol):_____

Functional Status:_____

     ADLs:_____

     IADLs:_____

Patient's Goals:_____

Gross Review of Systems:

Cardiovascular System: HR_____ RR_____ BP_____

Integumentary System: ❏ Not Impaired ❏ Impaired_____

_____

Neuromuscular System: ❏ Not Impaired ❏ Impaired_____

_____

Musculoskeletal System: ❏ Not Impaired ❏ Impaired_____

_____

Communication/Affect/Cognition: ❏ Not Impaired ❏ Impaired_____

_____

Tests and Measurements:

Aerobic Capacity/Endurance:

Test Performed:_____ Results:_____

_____

Test Performed:_____ Results:_____

_____

Girth:

Landmark	Right	Left
_____	____	____
_____	____	____
_____	____	____

Circulation:

Pulse(s)	Right	Left
_____	____	____
_____	____	____

Cranial/Peripheral Nerve Integrity:

Test:_____ Results:_____

_____

Test:_____ Results:_____

_____

Test:_____ Results:_____

_____

Gait/Locomotion/Balance:
Gait:_____

Transfers:_____

Bed Mobility:_____

Other functional mobility:_____

Integumentary Condition:
Location of wound:_____
Appearance of wound:_____
Size:_____ Odor:_____ Drainage:_____
Tunneling: _____ Periwound area:_____

ROM:

AROM	Joint:	Right	Left
	_____	_____	_____
	_____	_____	_____
	_____	_____	_____
	_____	_____	_____
	_____	_____	_____

PROM	Joint:	Right	Left
	_____	_____	_____
	_____	_____	_____
	_____	_____	_____
	_____	_____	_____
	_____	_____	_____

Strength:	Joint:	Right	Left
	_____	_____	_____
	_____	_____	_____
	_____	_____	_____
	_____	_____	_____
	_____	_____	_____

Posture: _____
_____

Flexibility:	Joint:	Right	Left
	_____	_____	_____
	_____	_____	_____
	_____	_____	_____
	_____	_____	_____
	_____	_____	_____

Reflexes: Reflex   Right   Left

—————————   ————   ————
—————————   ————   ————
—————————   ————   ————

Special Tests: Test: Right   Left

—————————   ————   ————
—————————   ————   ————
—————————   ————   ————
—————————   ————   ————
—————————   ————   ————

Intervention (Including patient education and HEP):

_____
_____
_____
_____
_____
_____

Assessment:

Physical therapy diagnosis:_____
_____
Prognosis:_____
Skilled services aimed at:_____
_____

Problem List:

Impairments: Functional Limitations:

———————————————   ———————————————
———————————————   ———————————————
———————————————   ———————————————
———————————————   ———————————————
———————————————   ———————————————

Anticipated Goals (STGs):

_____
_____
_____
_____
_____

Expected Outcomes (LTGs):

_____
_____
_____
_____
_____
_____

Plan (Including description of interventions, expected frequency and duration of services, and ultimate plan for discharge):

_____
_____
_____
_____
_____
_____
_____
_____
_____
_____
_____
_____
_____

_____

Therapist's Signature   **Date**

KNEE EVALUATION FORM

Anytown Physical Therapy and Rehabilitation
1000 Main St. Anytown, PA 15000

Knee Examination

Patient Name: _____ Age: _____ Sex: _____ Date: _____
Sport(s)/Occupation: _____ School/Employer: _____
Physician Hx: _____ Next Dr. Visit: _____
Dx/Surgical Procedure: _____ Date of Surgery: _____
Treatment Requested/Special Precautions: _____

Subjective:

Injured Knee: Right Left   *Dominant Leg:* Right Left
Onset: Acute Chronic   Date of Injury: _____
History/Mechanism: _____
_____
_____

Previous injury: Yes No   Similar Injury: Yes   No
Prior Treatment: _____
Chief Complaint: _____

ADL Limitations: ❏ Stairs   ❏ Uneven Ground   ❏ Squatting   ❏ Driving

                    ❏ Walking   ❏ Work/household/recreation activities

                    ❏ Other_____

X-rays/MRI:_____ Pain Rating (0-10):_____ Rest:_____
Activity:_____ Location:_____
Better: _____ Worse: _____
Numbness/Tingling? Yes   No   Where:_____ Global Rating(0-100):_____
Does Knee? Catch/ Pop (Y / N) Give-Way (Y / N) Swell (Y / N)   Sublux/Dislocate (Y / N)
Orthotics/Sleeves: _____ Injections (Y/N) #_____ Last:_____
PMH/Prior Surgeries:_____
Meds:_____
Hobbies/Activities/Work Duties:_____
Pt. Goals:_____
Other:_____

Objective:

General Observations: _____
Discoloration: ❏ Yes ❏ No   Where:_____
Swelling/Effusion: None   Minimal(1+)   Moderate(2+)   Severe(3+)
Where:_____
Skin Temperature (Circle):   Normal   Warm   Cold
Patellar Position/Tracking:_____ Patellar Mobility (↑,N,↓): Sup ___ Inf_____ Lat____ Med____

AROM:	Right	Left	*PROM:*	Right	Left	*Strength:*	Right	Left
Hip Flexion	____	____		____	____		____	____
Knee ROM	____	____		____	____		____	____
Ankle DF/PF	____	____		____	____		____	____
Ankle IV/EV	____	____		____	____		____	____

Gait: _____

    Assistive Device: None   Crutches   Cane   Walker   Other:_____

    Weight bearing status: NWB   PWB (_____%) FWB

Palpation: _____

_____

Girth Measurements:	Right	Left	Units (Circle):	cm	in
____Below	_____	_____			
____MJL	_____	_____			
____Above	_____	_____			
____Above	_____	_____			
____Above	_____	_____			

Functional Strength:	Right	Left
Quad Set	_____	_____
Flexion SLR	_____	_____
Extensor Lag	yes (_____°) no	yes (_____°) no

Special Tests:

Ant. Drawer:	L ____	R ____	Post. Drawer:	L ____	R ____
Lachman's:	L ____	R ____	Pivot Shift:	L ____	R ____
Valgus (0°):	L ____	R ____	Valgus (30°):	L ____	R ____
Varus (0°):	L ____	R ____	Varus (30°):	L ____	R ____
McMurray (IR):L ____		R ____	McMurray(ER):L ____		R ____
Apprehension:	L ____	R ____	Apley Compr:	L ____	R ____
Post. Sag:	L ____	R ____	Noble Compr:	L ____	R ____

    Other: _____

Flexibility:

Prone Quad:	L ____	R ____	ITB:	L ____	R ____
Hams:	L ____	R ____	Gastrocs:	L ____	R ____
Thomas Hip Flexor:	L ____	R ____			

    Other: _____

Neurovascular Tests: Sensation: _____   Capillary Refill: L _____   R _____

    Patellar Reflex: L _____   R _____   Achilles Reflex: L _____   R _____

Biomechanical Screen: _____

Leg Length: L ____   R ____   Short Leg: Right   Left   Symmetrical

Single Leg Stance (eyes open / closed):   L ____ seconds   R ____ seconds

Other: _____

Other Objective Tests/Measurements:

_____

_____

_____

_____

_____

_____

Treatment: _____Ice _____E –Stim _____US / Phono _____Russian

      _____Biofeedback (___uV) _____Whirlpool (Cold/Warm/Contrast)

      _____Ionto (Dex   Lidocaine   Other:_____)

#1   Parameters:_____

      Time:_____minutes

#2   Parameters:_____

      Time:_____minutes

      Other (Pat. Mobs/Stretching):_____

HEP Instruction and Performance (Time_____minutes):

_____ Quad Sets	_____ Glute Sets	_____ Heel Slides	_____ Seated Flexion
_____ HC Stretch	_____ HS Stretch	_____ Quad Stretch	_____ Hip Flex Stretch
_____ ITB Stretch	_____ Pat. Mobs	_____ Heel Props	_____ Mini-Squats
_____ Wall Squats	_____ Heel Raises	_____ Nose Touches	_____ Step-ups
_____SLR's (F, E, Abd, Add)		_____ (S,M,L) Tubing SLR's (F, E, Abd, Add)	

Other: _____

Evaluation/Plan of Care:

*PT Diagnosis:*_____

Problem List:

Impairments:

❏ Pain   ❏ Decreased Patellar Mobility

❏ Decreased ROM   ❏ Decreased LE Flexibility

❏ Decreased Strength ❏ Poor LE Biomechanics

❏ Swelling/Effusion   ❏ Decreased Balance

❏ Dependence with HEP

Other: _____

Functional Limitations:

❏ Gait/Stair Mobility

❏ Uneven terrain

❏ Squatting

❏ Work/recreation IADL's

❏ Driving

Other:_____

Short Term Goals (Time Frame _____ weeks / visits):

_____

_____

_____

_____

_____

Long Term Goals (Time Frame _____ weeks / visits):

_____

_____

_____

_____

Safety precautions/risk factors/barriers to D/C: _____

Rehab Potential/Prognosis: ❏ Good   ❏ Fair   ❏ Poor

Treatment: _____

Frequency: _____   *Duration:* _____

Therapist: _____   Date: _____

SHOULDER EVALUATION FORM

Anytown Physical Therapy and Rehabilitation
1000 Main St. Anytown, PA 15000

Shoulder Examination

Patient Name: _____ Age: _____ Sex: _____ Date: _____

Sport(s)/Occupation: _____ School/Employer: _____

Physician Hx: _____ Next Dr. Visit: _____

Dx/Surgical Procedure: _____ Date of Surgery: _____

Treatment Requested/Special Precautions: _____

Subjective:

Injured Shoulder: Right   Left   *Handedness:*   Right   Left

Onset: Acute   Chronic   Date of Injury: _____

History/Mechanism: _____

_____

Previous injury: ❏ Yes ❏ No

Similar Injury: ❏ Yes ❏ No

Prior Treatment: _____

Chief Complaint: _____

ADL Limitations:

❏ Carrying/lifting/reaching   ❏ Grooming/dressing   ❏ Work/recreation ADL's

❏ Household duties   ❏ Driving   ❏ Reading

❏ Sleeping   ❏ Other: _____

Pain Rating (0-10): _____ Rest: _____ Activity: _____ Location: _____

Better: _____ Worse: _____

Numbness/Tingling? Yes   No   Where: _____ Global Rating (0-

100): _____

Does Shoulder? Grind (Yes / No)   Click/Pop (Yes / No)   Come out of jt. (Yes / No)

Meds: _____ X-rays/MRI: _____

Slings/Supports: _____ Injections (Y/N) #_____ Last: _____

PMH/Prior Surgeries: _____

Hobbies/Activities/Work Duties: _____

Pt. Goals: _____

Objective:

General Observations: _____

Posture: ❏ Forward Head   ❏ Rounded Shoulders ❏ Kyphosis   ❏ Scoliosis

Scapular Winging: Left   Yes / No   Right   Yes / No

Scapular Rhythm: ❏ Normal ❏ Dyskinetic Functional Screen: Cervical Clearance: + / -

Back Scratch: Right _____ Left _____   Back Pat: Right _____ Left _____

Painful Arc: Yes / No   Where: _____° to _____°

AROM:	Right	Left	*PROM:*	Right	Left	*Strength:*	Right	Left
Sh Flexion	____	____	Sh Flexion	____	____	Sh Flexion	____	____
Sh ER(___°)	____	____	Sh ER(___°)	____	____	Sh ER(___°)	____	____
Sh IR (___°)	____	____	Sh IR (___°)	____	____	Sh IR (___°)	____	____
Sh Abd.	____	____	Sh Abd.	____	____	Sh Abd.	____	____
Sh Ext.	____	____	Sh Ext.	____	____	Sh Ext.	____	____
Elbow Flex.	____	____	Elbow Flex.	____	____	Elbow Flex.	____	____
Elbow Ext.	____	____	Elbow Ext.	____	____	Elbow Ext.	____	____

End Feel: ❏ Normal   ❏ Empty   ❏ Capsular/firm   Quality of Motion: _____

Sensation (↑, N, ↓):   Lt. Touch   Pin Prick

Myotomal Screen:

Cervical Rot (C1):	L ____ R ____	C2	L ____ R ____
Shoulder Elev (C2-4):	L ____ R ____	C3	L ____ R ____
Shoulder Abd. (C5):	L ____ R ____	C4	L ____ R ____
Elbow Flexion (C6):	L ____ R ____	C5	L ____ R ____
Wrist Ext. (C6):	L ____ R ____	C6	L ____ R ____
Elbow Ext. (C7):	L ____ R ____	C7	L ____ R ____
Wrist Flex. (C7):	L ____ R ____	C8	L ____ R ____
Thumb Ext. (C8):	L ____ R ____	T1	L ____ R ____
Finger Abd. (T1):	L ____ R ____		

Reflexes: Biceps: L ____ R ____   Brachioradialis: L ____ R ____
Triceps: L ____ R ____

Palpation: _____

Special Tests:

Empty Can:	L ____ R ____	Full Can:	L ____ R ____
Neer Impingement:	L ____ R ____	H-K Impinge:	L ____ R ____
AC Com/Dist:	L ____ R ____	S-C Stress:	L ____ R ____
Apprehension:	L ____ R ____	Relocation:	L ____ R ____
Sulcus:	L ____ R ____	O'Brien:	L ____ R ____
Ant./Post. Drawer:	L ____ R ____	Drop Arm:	L ____ R ____
Speed:	L ____ R ____	Clunk:	L ____ R ____
Adson's:	L ____ R ____	Roo's:	L ____ R ____

Other: _____

Scapular Evaluation: *Height of Scapula:*   L ____ R ____
SRM: Left + - Right + - SRT: Left + - Right + -
Modified Lat. Scap Slide (cm):

Position #1:	L ____ R ____	Position #2: L ____ R ____
Position #3:	L ____ R ____	Position #4: L ____ R ____

Flexibility:

Post. Cuff /Capsule: L ____ R ____	Scalenes:	L ____ R ____
SCM: L ____ R ____	Pec Minor:	L ____ R ____
Pec Major: L ____ R ____	Lats:	L ____ R ____

Other: _____

Treatment: ____Ice ____Moist Heat ____E–Stim ____US / Phono

____Combo ____Ionto (Dex Lidocaine MgSO$_4$ Other:_____)

#1 Parameters:_____

Time:_____minutes

#2 Parameters:_____

Time:_____minutes

Other(Jt. Mobs/Stretching):_____

_____

Postural Education: _____

_____

HEP Instruction and Performance (Time_____ minutes):

_____ PROM	_____ Wand AAROM	_____ Towel Slides
_____ Codman's	_____ Retractions	_____ Caudal Glides
_____ SB Stretch	_____ Cerv Flex Stretch	_____ Pit Checks
_____ Sleeper Stretch	_____ Pec Stretch	_____ Post. Caps. Stretch
_____ Serratus Punch	_____ Scap. Press ups	_____ Isometrics (IR, ER, F, E, Abd)
_____ (Y ,R, G, B) Tubing (IR, ER, F, E, Abd)		_____ Hughston's (#_____)
_____ Scapular Clock	_____ Scapular Prot/Retraction (seated/standing)	
_____ Standing Wt. Shifts	_____ Pulleys	_____ Thumb Tack Ex.
_____ Mass Mvmnts	_____ Push-up +	_____ "No Money" (0°, 90°, 180°)

Other Exercises: _____

Evaluation/Plan of Care:

*PT Diagnosis:*_____

Problem List:

Impairments: *Functional Limitations:*

❏ Pain	❏ Poor posture	❏ Reading ❏ Driving
❏ Decreased ROM	❏ Scapular dyskinesia	❏ Grooming/dressing
❏ Decreased strength	❏ Decreased joint mobility	❏ Carrying/lifting/reaching
❏ Decreased UE flexibility	❏ Dependence with HEP	❏ Work/household/rec. IADL's

Other: _____   Other: _____

Short Term Goals (Time Frame _____weeks/visits):

_____

_____

_____

_____

_____

Long Term Goals (Time Frame _____weeks/visits):

_____

_____

_____

_____

_____

Safety precautions/risk factors/barriers to D/C: _____

_____

_____

_____

Rehab Potential/Prognosis: ❑ Good ❑ Fair ❑ Poor

Treatment: ❑ Manual Therapy   ❑ Flexibility   ❑ Range of Motion Exercises

❑ Joint Mobilizations   ❑ Strengthening   ❑ Posture/Parascapular Training

❑ ADL/IADL Training   ❑ Scapular Taping   ❑ HEP Instruction/Progression

❑ Neuromuscular Reeducation ❑ Modalities to Decrease Pain/Spasm

❑ Other_____

_____

Frequency: _____ Duration: _____

Therapist: _____ Date: _____

References

1. Law M. *Evidence-Based Rehabilitation: A Guide to Practice*. Thorofare, NJ: SLACK Incorporated; 2002.

2. Nagi S. Disability concepts revisited: implications for prevention. In: Pope AM, Tarlov AR, eds. *Disability in America: Toward a national agenda for prevention*. Washington, DC: National Academy Press; 1991:309-327.

3. Quinn L, Gordon J. *Functional Outcomes: Documentation for Rehabilitation*. St. Louis, Mo: Saunders; 2003.

4. Fifty-Fourth World Health Assembly. *International Classification of Functioning, Disability and Health*. Geneva, Switzerland: World Health Organization; May 22, 2001. Report No.: WHA54.21.

5. World Health Organization. WHO publishes new guidelines to measure health [press release]. Geneva, Switzerland: World Health Organization; November 15, 2001.

6. World Health Organization. International classification of function. Available at: http://whqlib-doc.who.int/publications/2001/9241545429.pdf. Accessed June 18, 2004.

7. American Physical Therapy Association. *The Guide to Physical Therapist Practice*. Alexandria, Va: APTA; 2001.

8. Redgate N, Foto M. Pay by the rules: avoid Medicare audits and reduce payment denials with a sound strategy and proper documentation. *Physical Therapy Products*. 2003;October/November: 28-30.

9. American Physical Therapy Association House of Delegates. Principles for delivering physical therapy services within the health care system HOD 06-94-16-28. Available at: http://www.apta.org/governance/HOD/policies/HoDPolicies/Section_I/LEGISLATION/HOD_0 6941628. Accessed February 11, 2004.

10. Inaba M, Jones SL. Medical documentation for third-party payers. *Phys Ther*. 1977;57(7):791-794.

11. Reinstein L. Problem-oriented medical record: experience in 238 rehabilitation institutions. *Arch Phys Med Rehabil*. 1977;58(9):398-401.

12. Dinsdale SM, Mossman PL, Gullickson G, Anderson TP. The problem-oriented medical record in rehabilitation. *Arch Phys Med Rehabil*. 1970;51(8):488-492.

13. Milhous RL. The problem-oriented medical record in rehabilitation management and training. *Arch Phys Med Rehabil.* 1972;53(4):182-185.

14. Grabois M. The problem-oriented medical record: modification and simplification for rehabilitation medicine. *Southern Medical Journal.* 1977;70(11):1383-1385.

15. Reinstein LS. A rehabilitation evaluation system which complements the problem-oriented medical record. *Arch Phys Med Rehabil.* 1975;56(9):396-399.

16. Hebert LA. Basics of Medicare documentation for physical therapy. *Clinical Management in Physical Therapy.* 1981;1(3):13-14.

17. Baeten AM. Documentation: the reviewer perspective. *Topics in Geriatric Rehabilitation.* 1997;13(1):14-22.

18. Goode N. The reliable resource: physical therapy documentation. *PT—Magazine of Physical Therapy.* 1999;7(9):30-31.

19. Arriaga R. Liability awareness. Stories from the front: documentation and clinical decision making: a real-life scenario illustrates some basic risk-management principles. *PT—Magazine of Physical Therapy.* 2002;10(5):46-49.

20. Lewis K. Do the write thing: document everything. *PT—Magazine of Physical Therapy.* 2002;10(7):30-34.

21. Centers for Medicare and Medicaid Services. Centers for Medicare and Medicaid Services glossary. Available at: http://www.cms.hhs.gov/glossary. Accessed February 18, 2004.

22. Moorhead JF, Clifford J. Determining medical necessity of outpatient physical therapy services. *Am J Med Qual.* 1992;7(3):81-84.

23. Schunk CR. Liability awareness. Advice for the new physical therapist: here are some keys to avoiding risk once you've made the transition from student to practitioner. *PT—Magazine of Physical Therapy.* 2001;9(11):24-26.

24. Weed LL. *Medical Records, Medical Education, and Patient Care: The Problem-Oriented Medical Record as a Basic Tool.* Chicago: Year Book Medical Publishers; 1970.

25. Feinstein AR. The problems of the 'problem-oriented medical record'. *Ann Intern Med.* 1973;78(5):751-762.

26. Mcintyre N. The problem-oriented medical record. *BMJ.* 1973;2(5866):598-600.

27. White JA. Managing care. Documentation: making it meaningful. *Physical Therapy Case Reports.* 2000;3(2):78-79.

28. Clifton DW Jr. "Tolerated treatment well" may no longer be tolerated. *PT—Magazine of Physical Therapy.* 1995;3(10):24.

29. Abeln SH. Improving functional reporting (Utilization Review). *PT—Magazine of Physical Therapy.* 1996;4(3):26, 28-30.

30. Stamer MH. *Functional Documentation: A Process for the Physical Therapist.* Tucson, Ariz: Therapy Skill Builders; 1995.

31. Blecker D. Building better patient notes by using templates. *ACD-ASIM Observer.* 1998;18(9).

32. Feige M. Establishing standard rehabilitation evaluation forms. Arizona Association for Home Care. *Caring.* 1992;11(8):40-44.

33. Abeln SH. Liability awareness. Reporting risk check-up. *PT—Magazine of Physical Therapy.* 1997;5(10):38-42.

34. Brimer M. Focus on technology: making the move to electronic documentation. *PT—Magazine of Physical Therapy.* 1998;6(10):58-62.

35. American Physical Therapy Association. APTA connect. Available at: http://www.apta.org/PT_Practice/For_Clinicians/aptaconnect. Accessed June 14, 2004.

36. Ravitz KS. The HIPAA privacy final modified rule. *PT—Magazine of Physical Therapy.* 2002;10(11):21-25.

37. American Physical Therapy Association. States that permit physical therapy practice without a referral. Available at: http://www.apta.org/Govt_Affairs/state/directaccess/State3. Accessed May 27, 2004.

38. American Physical Therapy Association Board of Directors. Direction and supervision of the physical therapist assistant [RC 10-04]. Available at: http://apta.org/documents/membersonly/governance/2004draftPacket/RC10-04.pdf. Accessed May 27, 2004.

39. American Physical Therapy Association House of Delegates. Direction and supervision of the physical therapist assistant HOD 06-00-16-27. Available at: http://apta.org/governance/HOD/policies/HoDPolicies?Section_I/PRACTICE/HOD_06001627. Accessed May 27, 2004.

40. American Physical Therapy Association. *A normative model for PTA education.* Alexandria, Va: APTA; 1999.

41. American Physical Therapy Association House of Delegates. Standards of ethical conduct for the physical therapist assistant HOD 06-00-13-24. Available at: http://www.apta.org/PT_Practice/ethics_pt/ethics_pt_assistant. Accessed June 20, 2004.

42. Scholey ME. Documentation: a means of professional development... in physiotherapy. *Physiotherapy.* 1985;71(6):276-278.

43. Kettenbach G. *Writing SOAP Notes.* 2nd ed. Philadelphia, Pa: F.A. Davis; 1995.

44. American Physical Therapy Association. Reimbursement. Available at: http://www.apta.org/reimb. Accessed May 11, 2004.

45. American Physical Therapy Association. *The Reimbursement Resource Guide.* Alexandria, Va: APTA; 2002.

46. Centers for Medicare and Medicaid Services. CMS / HCFA history. Available at: http://www.cms.hhs.gov/about/history/. Accessed May 19, 2004.

47. CMS Press Office. The New Centers for Medicare and Medicaid Services [press release]. June 14, 2001.

48. U.S. Department of Health and Human Services. Medicare and You 2004. Available at: http://www.medicare.gov/Publications/Pubs/pdf/10050.pdf. Accessed May 19, 2004.

49. CMS Division of Institutional Claims Processing. Definition and uses of health insurance prospective payment system codes (HIPPS Codes). Available at: http://www.cms.hhs.gov/providers/hippscodes/hippsuses.pdf. Accessed May 24, 2004.

50. Centers for Medicare and Medicaid Services. MDS 2.0 - Manuals and forms. Available at: http://www.cms.hhs.gov/medicaid/mds20/man-form.asp. Accessed May 24, 2004.

51. Centers for Medicare and Medicaid Services. Inpatient rehab prospective payment system. Available at: http://www.cms.hhs.gov/providers/irfpps/. Accessed May 24, 2004.

52. Centers for Medicare and Medicaid Services. OASIS overview. Available at: http://www.cms.hhs.gov/oasis/hhoview.asp#B. Accessed May 25, 2004.

53. Centers for Medicare and Medicaid Services. Welcome to Medicaid. Available at: http://www.cms.hhs.gov/medicaid/. Accessed May 19, 2004.

54. Centers for Medicare and Medicaid Services. Beneficiary notices initiative. Available at: http://www.cms.hhs.gov/medicare/bni/. Accessed May 25, 2004.

55. Cohn R. Understanding insurance coverage. *PT—Magazine of Physical Therapy.* 1999;7(10).

56. NILS Insource. CCH insurance services glossary. Available at: http://insource.nils.com/gloss/GlossaryTerm.asp?tid=5713.

57. United Government Services L. Best documentation: concise and complete. Presented at: Medicare Outpatient Therapy Services Educational Seminar; May 17, 2004; Flatwoods, WVa.

58. Office of Civil Rights. Summary of the HIPAA privacy rule. Available at: http://www.os.dhhs.gov/ocr/privacysummary.pdf. Accessed June 24, 2004.

59. Office of Civil Rights. HIPAA fact sheet. Available at: http://www.hhs.gov/news/facts/privacy.html. Accessed May 28, 2004.

60. American Medical Association. AMA Opinions and standards: 5.07 Confidentiality: Computers. Available at: http://www.netreach.net/~wmanning/ama507.htm. Accessed May 28, 2004.

61. American Physical Therapy Association Ethics and Judicial Committee. Guide for conduct for the physical therapist assistant. Available at: http://www.apta.org/PT_Practice/ethics_pt/affiliate_conuct. Accessed June 20, 2004.

62. Centers for Medicare and Medicaid Services. Fraud overview. Available at: http://www.medicare.gov/FraudAbuse/Overview.asp. Accessed June 24, 2004.

63. Price SA. Risk Management. Presented at: West Virginia Physical Therapy Association Chapter Meeting; August 9, 1997; Flatwoods, WVa.

64. Smith LC. Risk management: the hot topics. *PT—Magazine of Physical Therapy.* 2000;8(12):26-33.

65. Agency for Healthcare Research and Quality. Making health care safer: a critical analysis of patient safety practices. Available at: http://www.ahrq.gov/clinic/ptsafety/ . Accessed June 25, 2004.

66. Federation of State Boards of Physical Therapy. A model practice act for physical therapy. Available at: http://fsbpt.org/publications/index.asp. Accessed June 20, 2004.

67. American Physical Therapy Association House of Delegates. Documentation authority for physical therapy services HOD 06-00-20-05. Available at: http://apta.org/governance/HOD/policies/HoDPolicies/Section_I/PRACTICE/HOD_06002005. Accessed September 6, 2004.

Index

WAIT

...There's More!

SLACK Incorporated's Professional Book Division offers a wide selection of products in the field of Physical Therapy. We are dedicated to providing important works that educate, inform, and improve the knowledge of our customers. Don't miss out on our other informative titles that will enhance your collection.

The PTA Handbook: Keys to Success in School and Career for the Physical Therapist Assistant
Kathleen Curtis, PhD, PT and Peggy DeCelle Newman, PT, MHR
328 pp., Soft Cover, 2005, ISBN 1-55642-621-6
Order #46216, **$34.95**

The PTA Handbook: Keys to Success in School and Career for the Physical Therapist Assistant contains extensive coverage of the most pertinent issues for the physical therapist assistant, including the physical therapist-physical therapist assistant preferred relationship, evidence-based practice and problem-solving, essentials of information competence, and diversity.

Quick Reference Dictionary for Physical Therapy, Second Edition
Jennifer Bottomley, PhD^2, MS, PT
624 pp., Soft Cover, 2003, ISBN 1-55642-580-5
Order #45805, **$28.95**

Physical Therapist Assistant Exam Review, Fourth Edition
Theresa Meyer, PT
336 pp., Soft Cover, 2000, ISBN 1-55642-589-9
Order #45899, **$27.95**

Patient Practitioner Interaction: An Experiential Manual for Developing the Art of Health Care, Third Edition
Carol M. Davis, EdD, PT
352 pp., Soft Cover, 1998, ISBN 1-55642-400-0
Order #44000, **$35.95**

Complementary Therapies in Rehabilitation: Evidence for Efficacy in Therapy, Prevention, and Wellness, Second Edition
Carol M. Davis, EdD, PT, MS, FAPTA
416 pp., Hard Cover, 2004, ISBN 1-55642-581-3
Order #45813, **$44.95**

PT Study Cards in a Box
Theresa Meyer, PT
288 Study Cards, 2001, ISBN 1-55642-482-5
Order #44825, **$50.95**

Quick Reference Neuroscience for Rehabilitation Professionals: The Essential Neurologic Principles Underlying Rehabilitation Practice
Sharon A. Gutman, PhD, OTR
288 pp., Soft Cover, 2001, ISBN 1-55642-463-9
Order #34639, **$38.95**

Practical Kinesiology for the Physical Therapist Assistant
Jeff G. Konin, PhD, AT, PT
240 pp., Soft Cover, 1999, ISBN 1-55642-299-7
Order #42997, **$38.95**

Special Tests for Orthopedic Examination, Second Edition
Jeff G. Konin, PhD, AT, PT; Denise Wiksten, PhD, ATC; Jerome A. Isear, Jr., MS, PT, ATC-L; and Holly Brader, MPH, ATC, CHES
352 pp., Soft Cover, 2002, ISBN 1-55642-591-0
Order #45910, **$36.95**

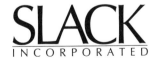